STUDY GUIDE

To Accompany

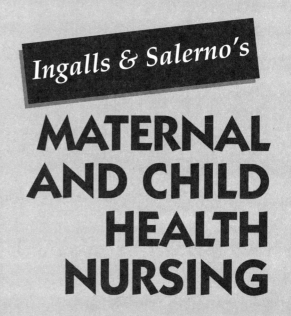

Ingalls & Salerno's

MATERNAL AND CHILD HEALTH NURSING

Children learn what they live

If a child lives with criticism,
He learns to condemn.
If a child lives with hostility,
He learns to fight.
If a child lives with ridicule,
He learns to be shy.
If a child lives with shame,
He learns to feel guilty.
If a child lives with tolerance,
He learns to be patient.
If a child lives with encouragement,
He learns confidence.
If a child lives with praise,
He learns to appreciate.
If a child lives with fairness,
He learns justice.
If a child lives with security,
He learns to have faith.
If a child lives with approval,
He learns to like himself.
If a child lives with acceptance and friendship,
He learns to find love in the world.

Dorothy Law Nolte

STUDY GUIDE
To Accompany

Ingalls & Salerno's

MATERNAL AND CHILD HEALTH NURSING

A. Joy Ingalls, R.N., M.S.
Former Instructor, Maternal and Child Health Nursing,
Grossmont Vocational Nursing Program,
Grossmont Health Occupations Center, Santee, California

M. Constance Salerno, R.N., M.S., P.N.P.
Professor Emeritus of Child Health Nursing
San Diego State University, San Diego, California

SIXTH EDITION

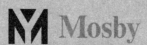

St. Louis Baltimore Boston Carlsbad Chicago Naples New York Philadelphia
London Madrid Mexico City Singapore Sydney Tokyo Toronto Wiesbaden

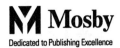

Mosby

Dedicated to Publishing Excellence

A Times Mirror Company

Editor: Susan Epstein
Senior Developmental Editor: Beverly J. Copland
Production Editor: Rick Dudley

SIXTH EDITION

Printed in the United States of America

Composition by AlphaByte & Co.
Printing/binding by Plus Communications

Mosby–Year Book, Inc.
11830 Westline Industrial Drive
St. Louis, Missouri 63146

95 96 97 98 99 / 9 8 7 6 5 4 3 2 1

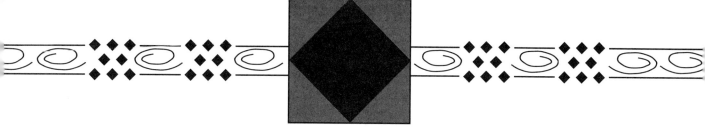

Preface

The sixth edition of this Study Guide, while maintaining the basic structure of its immediate predecessor, reflects changes in content found in its parent publication, the eighth edition of the text, *Maternal and Child Health Nursing.*

Each exercise begins with an introductory statement and clinical tie-in questions that seek to initiate exploration and analysis of certain features of the students' assigned clinical setting or community. Each chapter contains study questions of various types: fill-in, short answer, or matching exercises. Most exercises also contain questions related to specific clinical situations. At the end of each exercise, optional "probe questions," with a suggested bibliography, are included for special study or make-up assignments. Answers to the study questions found in each chapter are at the back of the guide. As in the past the pages of the text where answers may be found are indicated in the margins next to the questions.

We hope the guide continues to be an asset to the student and teacher participating in the care of the child and family. It is designed to assist in both review and continued investigation of this extensive and interesting field.

We are indebted to many students, teaching colleagues, physicians, nurses, and patients who over the years have aided in this endeavor. We recognize the welcome assistance of the capable writers of the revision of the text upon which this Study Guide is based. We also want to express our sincere appreciation to our hard working editor Susan Epstein and Senior Developmental Editor Beverly Copland and to the staff who have helped bring this edition to the printed page.

A. Joy Ingalls
M. Constance Salerno

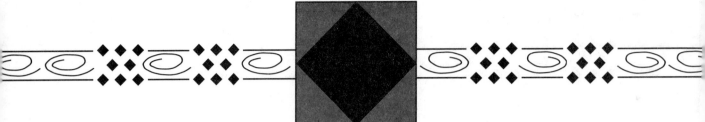

Suggestions to Students

This Study Guide has been prepared to help you identify some of the significant aspects of perinatal and pediatric nursing, to provide methods of evaluation and review, and to stimulate additional reading and investigation in the field. Each exercise contains both subjective and objective items, based on material presented in the eighth edition of the text *Maternal and Child Health Nursing*. The exercises in the Study Guide correspond to units in the text.

If you study and respond to the questions in each exercise, you should meet most learning objectives for the theory portion of many maternal and child nursing courses designed for the first-level, bedside nurse. Study questions include: fill-in, true or false, matching, and analysis of clinical situations. All exercises include one answer multiple choice questions. An answer key at the back of the Study Guide supplies answers to the study questions. For reference to the text the page numbers containing the material have been placed next to the questions. A list of commonly misspelled words in charting can be found in the appendix.

The clinical tie-ins found near the beginning of each exercise are included to emphasize the relationship between theory and practice; that is, between textual material and the students' involvement in the clinical situation. Selected tie-ins may be chosen for personal investigation or report. The probe questions at the end of each exercise are designed to allow the student to pursue a particular topic with an introductory list of special reading selections.

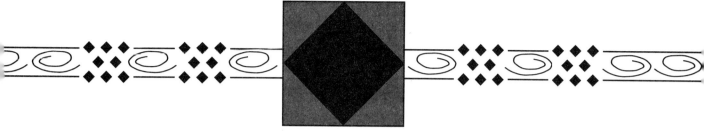

Contents

viii Contents

STUDY GUIDE

To Accompany

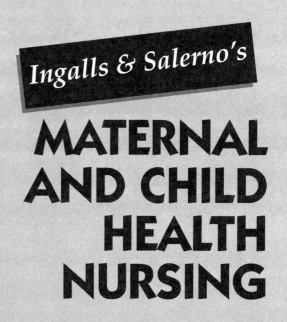

Ingalls & Salerno's

MATERNAL
AND CHILD
HEALTH
NURSING

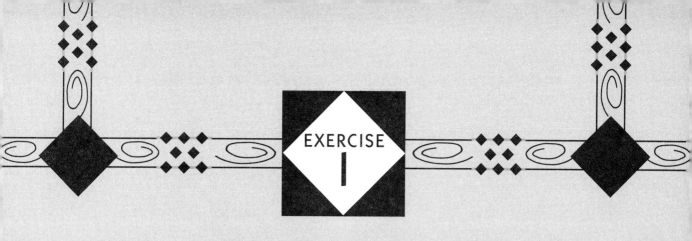

PERSPECTIVES IN MATERNAL AND CHILD HEALTH NURSING

It is essential that nurses have some understanding of the development of maternal and child health care through the years so they can appreciate the progress that has been made, as well as the problems of the present. It is also appropriate that they consider some of the basic methods and developing concepts, organizational structures, standards, and expanding roles used to identify, guide, and provide nursing care in all areas of practice. Nurses also must continue to learn more about the populations they serve and the dynamics of family stability and change. Now, as never before, we as a nation must seek viable answers to the many challenges to individual, family, and community health. We all must nurture a commitment to deliver the best care possible to all our citizens, infants to elders.

CLINICAL TIE-IN

1. Have you, your relatives, or friends known a woman who died in childbirth? Have you personally known of an infant who died within the first month of life? If so, what were the contributing causes?
2. Talk to a woman whose children were born in a hospital during the 1960s or 1970s. How was her maternity care organized? How long was her hospitalization after birth? What does she think was good about her experience? What does she recall that she wished she could have changed?
3. What types of maternity services do hospitals in your community provide? (Examples may be departmentalized care with separate labor, delivery, postpartum, and nursery areas; birthing rooms; single room maternity care; rooming-in; "couplet care".) Do you know any mothers who have had a planned birth at home?
4. What is the average cost of private prenatal care and delivery in a hospital setting in your community? What insurance coverage currently is available? What coverage do local health maintenance organizations (HMOs) provide? Are you aware if there are many local women who are not receiving adequate prenatal care?
5. List the resources in your community that provide financial or other assistance to needy mothers and children. How is eligibility determined?
6. Interview a practicing clinical nurse specialist, perinatal or pediatric nurse practitioners, or certified nurse midwife. What are his/her responsibilities and scope of practice? How many clients are they serving? What kind of patients are being seen?

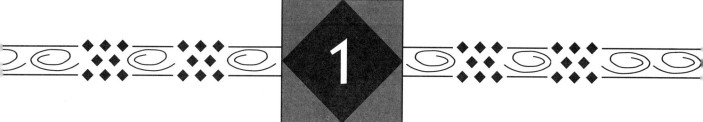

History and Current Trends in Maternal and Child Health Nursing

Page Reference

1. Match the medical or nursing pioneer in the right column with a contribution to maternal/child health care with which they have been associated. Use each letter only once.

4	_e_ Confirmed that puerperal fever was caused by bacteria	a. Joseph Lister
5	_b_ Helped to establish the Henry St. Settlement House, visiting nurse and school nurse services	b. Lillian Wald
		c. Ignaz Semmelweis
		d. Florence Nightingale
4	_f_ Founded first pediatric clinic in the U.S.A.	e. Louis Pasteur
4	_c_ Taught that puerperal fever was spread by unwashed hands	f. Abraham Jacobi
		g. Margaret Sanger
5	_h_ Advocated nurse midwifery in the U.S.A.	h. Mary Breckenridge
4	_A_ Called "Father of Antisepsis"	
5	_g_ Organized family planning centers	
5	_d_ Formed historical basis for nursing's role in health promotion	

2. Fill in the following blanks highlighting past to present federal involvement in promoting maternal and child health. Usually held at the beginning of each

5   decade from 1901-1971 the [a] _____ White

_____ house conference _____ focused on the needs of children and youth throughout the United States. Largely because of problems associated with the use of children in the nation's labor force, the

6   [b] _____Children's Bureau_____ was founded in 1912. Studies by this federal agency revealed high maternal and infant mortality rates among the poor. From 1935 to the present, various governmental attempts have been made to provide more health care services to needy families, mothers,

6   and children, by the enactment of [c] _Social Security Legislation_.

Among the health care services provided with the Social Security Act (SSA) are: (mention four)

6   [d] _Foster care_

Family Planning

Education of public health personnel

Medicaid

A program specifically designed to aid preschool children from disadvantaged

6   backgrounds founded in 1965 is [e] _Project Head Start_.

WIC or [f] _Special Supplement Food Program for women, Infants and children_ helps pregnant women and new mothers and their children up to age 5 years. Other more recent federal agencies created are:

7   [g] 1978 _National Center of Child Abuse_

7   [h] 1982 _Missing Childrens Act_

3.   List two United Nations' sponsored organizations that have been particularly involved in the international promotion of maternal and child health:

7   [a] _UNICEF - United Nations Childrens fund_

7   [b] _WHO - World health organization_

9   4.   Define the following frequently used statistics by placing the proper letter next to the descriptive phrase.

_e_	Number of deaths from birth to 19 years of age per 100,000 population for that age group	a. Infant mortality
_d_	Number of maternal deaths per 100,000 live births	b. Birth rate
_a_	The number of children per 1000 live births who die before their first birthday	c. Neonatal mortality
_b_	Number of live births per 1000 population	d. Maternal mortality
_c_	Number of infant deaths that occur in the first 28 days of life per 1000 births	e. Childhood mortality

10   5. The maternal mortality rate in the United States steadily declined to a low of

[a] _____7.3_____ in 1990. The four leading causes of maternal death are:

[b] _Pulomonary embolisim_

[c] _PIH Pregnancy Induced hypertension_

[d] _Ectopic Pregnancy_

[e] _Hemmorrahage_

10   6. The infant mortality rate in the United States for the year 1990 was

[a] _____9.2_____. This rate was greater than that of 21 other nations in the world. Origins of this poor ranking may be traced partially to

[b] _Lack of access to prenatal care_ and the [c] _High rate of adolscent pregnnc_

The leading causes of infant mortality in the United States are:

[d] _Low birth weight_

[e] _Birth defects_

[f] _Sudden Infant Death Syndrome_

Low birth weight is defined as under [g] _____5.8 lbs_ or [h] _2500 gram_

Prematurity or preterm birth is defined as [i] _Birth before 38 weeks gestat_

12   7. List the three broad national health objectives for the year 2000 that have been iden-tified by the U.S. Department of Health and Human Services. If implemented, they should impact all stages of American life.

[a] _Increase the span of healthy life for all Americans_

[b] _Decrease health departies among Americans_

[c] _Achieve access to preventive Services for Americons_

5   8. The greatest improvement in maternal morbidity and mortality rates in the early 1900s resulted from the
    a. Increase in the number of obstetricians
    b. Prenatal care given by physicians and nurses ✓
    c. Availability of antibiotics and other new drugs
    d. Ability to administer blood transfusions

4   9. By the 1900s as the threat of hospital infection in the United States receded and tech-nologies expanded:
    a. The old role of the midwife was enlarged
    b. Maternity care became less expensive
    c. Family involvement in labor and delivery increased
    d. Home births became the exception ✓

4   10.   In the late 1960s, growing dissatisfaction with hospital-based maternity experiences initiated a broad long-lasting consumer-orientated emphasis most often termed the:
               a.   Natural childbirth movement
               b.   Pregnant Patient's Bill of Rights
               c.   Lamaze Method
               d.   Psychoprophylactic Approach

8   11.   The current practices of early discharge, regionalization of services, and establishment of a pretreatment payment system based on diagnosis (DRG) are all methods used primarily to:
               a.   Encourage better record keeping
               b.   Reduce health care costs
               c.   Promote patient self-reliance
               d.   Avoid unnecessary family separation

9   12.   In maternal and child health care the focus is shifting to:
               a.   More simple therapeutic methods
               b.   Preventive perinatal and pediatric care
               c.   Full service capability at each health center
               d.   In-hospital rather than ambulatory care

10   13.   Many conditions and behaviors may lead to the birth of low birth weight infants, but studies indicate that the most powerful and pervasive factor is that of:
               a.   Drug abuse
               b.   Smoking
               c.   Malnutrition
               d.   Poverty

12   14.   After the age of 1 year, the leading cause of death throughout childhood is:
               a.   Infectious diseases
               b.   Accidents
               c.   Injuries
               d.   Homicide

9   15.   The demographic makeup of the population of the United States has always been in the process of change. If present trends continue, by the year 2000, all the observations below are expected to be true *EXCEPT*:
               a.   More women beginning child bearing after age 35
               b.   More adolescents 15-17 years of age
               c.   More older than younger children
               d.   A decrease in the non-Caucasian population

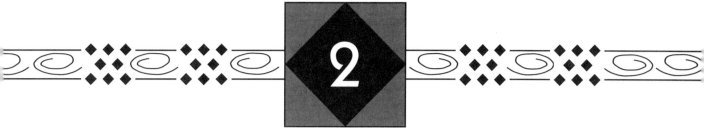

Contemporary Maternal and Child Health Nursing Practice

Page Reference

15

1. The ANA defines maternal and child health nursing (MCHN) as a

   [a] _Specialized_ area of nursing focused on the [b] _health needs_

   _____ and [c] _identifiable response for woman,_

   their partners and families to [d] _real or potential_ _____ health

   problems associated with [e] _childbearing & childrearing_ .

   It includes concern for the developing [f] _fetus_ from [g] _conception_

   to birth and the child from [h] _birth through adolescent_

15

2. The practice of maternal and child health nursing emphasizes

   [a] _health promotion_ _____

   and the [b] ___ _prevention_ _____ of disease.

16

3. Numerous types and levels of nursing and medical personnel participate in maternal and child health care. A number of nurses and physicians have received advanced preparation and have roles involving greater specialization and/or responsibility in their fields. Examples of such evolving roles would be:

   in nursing [a]   in medicine [b]

   _____   _____

   _____   _____

   _____   _____

17-18   4. List the five steps that typically make up the systematic circular problem-solving approach to clinical nursing care called the nursing process:

[a] _Assessment_

[b] _Nursing Diagnosis_

[c] _Planning_

[d] _Implementation_

[e] _Evaluation_

18-19   5. Two nursing organizations that have greatly influenced the development and definition of maternal and child health nursing are the:

[a] _The Division on Maternal & Child Health Nursing Practice_

[b] _The Association of Womens heaeth, Obstetric, Neonate_

18   6. The nursing standard of care is defined as the [a] _average_

degree of skill and care exhibited by a nurse with comparable

[b] _education_ in similar [c] _circumstances_ .

18   7. Three ways that nurses can reduce the risk of committing an error that violates the standard of care follow:

[a] _carefully documenting care in patient record_

[b] _obtaining informed consent_ to performing

any procedure; and [c] _pursuing continuing education_.

21   8. State the five basic ethical principles in health care:

[a] _____

[b] _____

[c] _____

[d] _____

[e] _Jus_ _____

16   9. The developing knowledge base that guides nursing practice has been organized around four major concepts or ideas. They are usually stated as:
a. Client, health, family, and nursing
b. Patient, illness, community, and care
c. Person, health, environment, and nursing
d. Individual, life process, prevention, and adaptability

16

10. Some health care settings have adopted certain perspectives or conceptual frameworks. When employed these models:
    a. Must be accepted by all caregivers without change
    b. May help shape client assessment, care, and documentation
    c. Are uniformly implemented by the nursing community
    d. Tend to limit the potential of the individual for change

17-18

11. When the expected outcomes of a patient's plan of care do not occur within a particular time frame, it may be that:
    a. Initial assessment information or nursing diagnosis was incorrect or incomplete
    b. Planned intervention and expectations were inappropriate, too optimistic, or poorly implemented
    c. Evaluation techniques were faulty
    d. Any part of, or combination of a, b, or c could contribute to failure to achieve the desired outcomes

18

12. Failing to meet the standard of care includes all of the following situations EXCEPT:
    a. Failing to prevent patient injury
    b. Failing to do something that should have been done
    c. Doing something incorrectly
    d. Doing something outside the scope of nursing practice

18

13. Nurses notes should document which responsibilities:
    a. Behavior observed
    b. Vital signs obtained
    c. Medications and treatment
    d. All of the above

20

14. The practice of "defensive health care":
    a. Is designed primarily to protect the patient
    b. Is accompanied by lower liability insurance premiums
    c. Is contributing to higher health care costs
    d. Is reduced by an increase in malpractice litigation

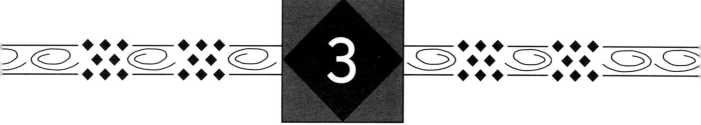

The Family in a Multicultural Society

Page Reference

24

1. "Family" may be defined various ways. Friedman's definition, broad enough to cover most of the varying family forms found in America today, is:

   two or more people who are joined together by bonds of sharing & emotional closeness; identifying themselves as family

24

2. Nurses should note that the above sociological explanation differs from the legal definition, which describes family as members:

   Members bound together by the civil or religious bonds of marriage and adoption

25

3. Describe the following family forms:

   a. Nuclear family *mother, father and dependant child or children*

   b. Nuclear dyad *mother, father, both head of household. with no children or mother father with adult children not living at home*

   c. Single-parent family *Mother or father, head of household with dependent Child or children*

   d. Three-generation extended family *nuclear familey, nuclear dyad, or single-parent family living with one or more parents in the same household.*

e.   Extended kin network _Two or more nuclear family living in close proximity and proving mutral support_

24

4.   In 1991 the U.S. Bureau of Census disclosed findings that the

[a] ___Traditional___ ___nuclear___ family structure was found in only 26% of all households. In the majority of households of this type both parents were employed. More than 60% of

employed married women had children under [b]___6___ years of age.

25

5.   The most rapidly growing family form is the _Single_

___parent___ family.

24

6.   Indicate four changes in attitudes and expectations concerning family life that have contributed to the decrease of the nuclear family in the United States as well as other changes in family structure and function since the 1950s:

[a] _increased acceptance & women's employment outside the hour_

[b] _more tolerance of homosexual relationship_

[c] _more tolerance of divorce_

[d] _marriage no longer view as healthy satisfying life style for rearing children_

26

7.   The text lists five major functions that continue to be the main responsibilities of the family and that help support the individual and the society.

a.   What are these functions?

(1) _Affective_

(2) _Reproductive_

(3) _Socialization_

(4) _Health care_

(5) _Economic Support_

b.   Thought question: Give two examples of functions formerly considered the exclusive domain of the family which today have largely been assumed by other social institutions.

Education — School

religious — church

24-29   8. A balance between the developmental needs of individuals in a family and the developmental tasks of the family unit is not always easy to achieve or maintain, especially if significant health problems are present. Consider a family you know that is undergoing the added stress of illness of a family member (adult or child). Maintaining anonymity, briefly describe the situation:

   a. Identify the family form.
   b. List the members of the family by sex and age.
   c. Note their individual development needs using the chart Stages and Developmental Tasks of the Individual's Psychosocial Development adapted from Erikson (see text p. 28).
   d. Identify the family's Life Cycle Stage as adapted from Duvall and Miller (see text p. 27).
   e. List the family's predominant developmental challenges adapted from Friedman (see text p. 29).
   f. Do the individuals in the family appear to be successful in meeting their respective psychosocial challenges?
   g. Does the family unit seem to be able to respond to the tasks of its stage of development?
   h. How do you think the presence of illness impacts each individual and the family as a whole?
   i. What kind of assistance would help ease the problems identified?
   j. How could a knowledgeable nurse help?

Students may find that making some type of chart may help organize their presentation. See chart.

PSYCHOSOCIAL CHALLENGES TO INDIVIDUAL FAMILY MEMBERS AND THE FAMILY UNIT					
(Create symbols ___ female; ___ male; Relationship M=mother; F=father; GP=grandparent, etc.)					
First name	Sex	Age	Relation	Individual stage of psychosocial development and primary challenge	Family life cycle stage and developmental tasks family form: _____

9. Vocabulary match

30   _2_ a. acculturation

30   _3_ b. stereotype

27   _1_ c. ethnocentrism

27   _5_ d. culture

27   _4_ e. ethnicity

30   _6_ f. egalitarian

(1) belief that values/practices of one's own culture are superior to all others
(2) process of adopting the values of the dominant culture
(3) labeling persons as group without accounting for individual differences
(4) sense of belonging to a particular group distinguished by culture, religion, language, race
(5) learned patterns of behavior shared by a specific group
(6) demonstrating a democratic perspective

27, 30 10. Cultural groups have been identified by their common values in five different areas affecting attitudes toward life. List the areas involved and at least one example of related patient perspectives or behaviors that influence health and health care providers.

[a] _____ / _____

_____

_____

[b] _____ / _____

_____

_____

[c] _____ / _____

_____

_____

[d] _____ / _____

_____

_____

[e] _____ / _____

_____

_____

11. Self-examination exercises

27, 30

    a.   How would you describe yourself regarding the attitudes reflected in the five value areas outlined in question 10?

_____

_____

_____

33

    b.   Using the Cultural Assessment Box in chapter 3, investigate your own cultural identity; write out an observation of yourself.

_____

_____

_____

33

    c.   Is it important that nurses be aware of their own beliefs, values, and practices? Why?

yes. So they will be more open to value those of other individuals

_____

23-25

12. Nurses working in perinatal or pediatric settings in the United States should develop some understanding of all of the following topics EXCEPT:
    a.   How families function and adapt
    b.   How culture may influence health practices
    c.   How family structure has been diversified
   ✓d.   How family functions have remained the same

24, 33

13. In contemporary America, the primary supportive function of the family has become:
    a.   Education
    b.   Economic
   ✓c.   Affection
    d.   Reproductive

24

14. Shifting attitudes and expectations involving the family have fostered all the developments below *EXCEPT*:
    a.   Decrease in family size
   ✓b.   Decrease in incidence of marriage
    c.   Increase in divorce rates
    d.   Increase of first births by older women

25   15. Single parent and minority families make up a disproportionate number of families that are:
     a.   Living at or below the poverty line
     b.   Lacking health insurance
     c.   Headed by women
     ✓d. All of the above

27   16. A nurse who believes lack of eye contact indicates dishonesty may have difficulty dealing with a client who is:
     a.   Irish
     b.   African-American
     c.   Asian
     d.   Native American

27, 30-33   17. Identifying differences in beliefs, values, and practices of a client from those of a nurse may assist the health care worker to avoid all of the following EXCEPT:
     a.   Ethnocentric behavior
     b.   Communication problems
     ✓c. Individualized care
     d.   Stereotyped responses

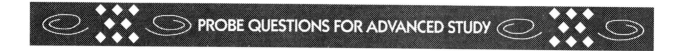

PROBE QUESTIONS FOR ADVANCED STUDY

1. What kinds of obstacles confronted Semmelweis and Holmes in the 1800s when they tried to prove that puerperal fever was spread by medical personnel?

REFERENCES

For the majority of students the most accessible, authoritative accounts of the problems faced by these medical pioneers (and others such as Louis Pasteur and Joseph Lister) are contained in standard encyclopedias available in public and school libraries. However, the references below have special merit.

Bendiner E:. Semmelweis, lone rager against puerperal fever, Hosp Prac 22(2):194-6+, 1987.

Larson E.: Innovations in health care: antisepsis as a case study, Am J Pub Health 79(1):92-9, 1989.

Thompson M: The cry and the covenant, Cutchogue, NY, 1991, Buccaneer Books.

Wertz RW and Wertz DC: Lying-in, a history of childbirth in America, New Haven, 1989, Yale University Press.

2. Certain functions and responsibilities previously thought to belong only to physicians are being given to advanced practice nurses such as the pediatric nurse practitioner. Discuss the role of pediatric nurse practitioners. What are their functions and responsibilities? Where do these nurses receive their educational preparation? How long are current courses of study? How well are they accepted by patients and physicians? How have they contributed to the health of children?

REFERENCES

Brown SA and Grimes DE: Nurse practitioners and certified nurse midwives: a meta-analysis on process of care, clinical outcomes and cost-effectiveness of nurses in primary care roles, Publ no NP-85 Washington, DC, 1993 American Nurses Association.

Jacox A: The OTA report: a policy analysis, Nurse Outlook 35(6):262-268, 1987.

Kalish PA and Kalish BJ: The advance of American nursing, Boston, 1986, Little, Brown & Co.

Morain C: On her own, RN 55(7):28-32, 1992.

Murphy MA: A brief history of pediatric nurse practitioners and NAP-NAP 1964-1990, J Pediatr Health Care 4(6):332-7, 1990.

O'Connor KS: Advanced practice nurses in an environment of health care reform MCN 19(2):65-68, 1994.

Robinson K: Selecting a pediatric nurse practitioner program, Pediatr Nurs 18(2):176-82, 1992.

3. In what ways are nurse-midwives contributing to maternal and child health in the United States? What types of preparation and legal status do they have? What do the initials CNM mean?

REFERENCES

Bell KE and Mills JI: Certified nurse midwife effectiveness in the health maintenance organization obstetric team, Obstetrics Gynecol 74(1):112-6, 1989.

Ericson D: So you want to be a midwife, Int J Childbirth Educ 5(3):17-18, 1990.

Jacox A: The OTA report: a policy analysis, Nurse Outlook 35(6):262-268, 1987.

Obstetrics—Midwifery in the 1990s, 1993 medical and health annual, Chicago, 1992, Encyclopedia Brittanica.

Rooks J and Haas JE eds: Nurse-midwifery in America, Washington, DC, 1986, American College of Nurse Midwives Foundation.

Rooks JP: Nurse midwifery: the window is wide open, Am J Nurs 90(12):30-36, 1990.

Stivers SR: A challenge to nurse-midwifery, J Nurse Midwifery 38(5):288-292, 1993.

U.S. Congress, Office of Technology Assessment: Nurse practitioners, physicians assistants and certified nurse midwives: a policy analysis, Washington, DC, 1986, U.S. Government Printing Office.

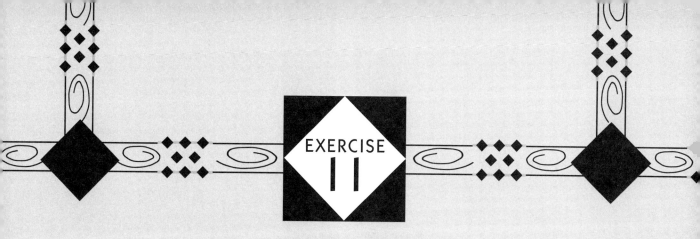

HUMAN REPRODUCTION

Student nurses must have a basic knowledge of human structure and function regardless of their current subject emphasis or clinical area assignment. In perinatal nursing, although all body systems are significant, reproductive anatomy and physiology are of paramount importance. The following questions and discussions are designed to review particularly those body features and mechanisms crucial to the creation of the next generation and to help students evaluate their understanding of this fascinating and sometimes controversial subject.

CLINICAL TIE-IN

1. Look at some prenatal records. Determine how the pelvic adequacy of your perinatal clients was evaluated. Attend, if possible, an ultrasound evaluation of uterine contents.

2. When performing a catheterization, checking an episiotomy, or assisting during a perineal repair, try to use the occasion for anatomical orientation.

3. Approximately how many of the postpartum mothers you have cared for had perineal incisions or episiotomies? Do you know why the incisions were made? What kind of extra care did they need? Did any of the women have perineal lacerations? Check their charts.

4. While caring for a postpartum mother, note the difference in the position of the uterine fundus and the contour of the lower abdominal wall (over the bladder) before and after she voids.

5. Among the mothers you have met during perinatal contacts, have any volunteered the information that although the current pregnancy is accepted, it was not planned?

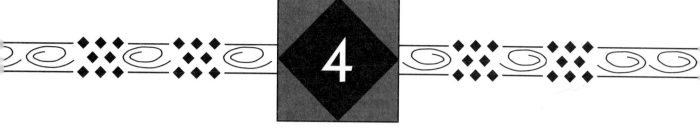

Female Reproductive System

Page Reference

A basic understanding of the female external and internal anatomy is essential to the nurse. Using Figs. 4-1, 4-2, and 4-3, identify all the lettered areas of the female anatomy. Describe the function or nursing significance of the anatomy indicated by the boldface letters and asterisks.

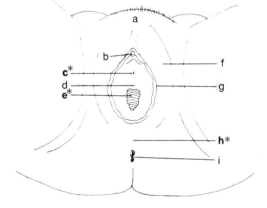

Fig. 4-1. Female external genitalia.

Page		
37-38	1. a.	_____
37-38	b.	_____
38	c.*	_____
38	d.	_____
39, 40, 42	e.*	_____
37, 38	f.	_____
38	g.	_____
38, 39	h.*	_____
38	i.	_____

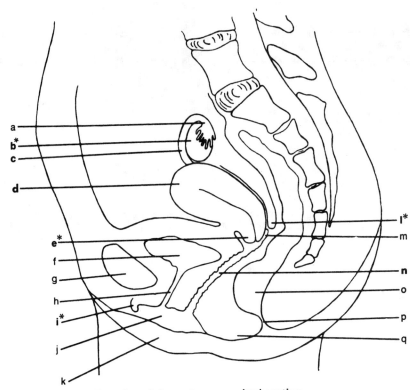

Fig. 4-2. Female pelvic anatomy, sagittal section.

37-38	2. a.	_____
38	b.*	_____
39-41	c.*	_____
40-41	d.*	_____
40-41	e.*	_____
39, 40	f.	_____
37, 38	g.	_____
38, 39	h.	_____
38	i.*	_____
38	j.	_____
38-39	k.	_____
39, 41-42	l.*	_____
39, 41	m.	_____
42	n.*	_____
39	o.	_____
38	p.	_____
38-39	q.	_____

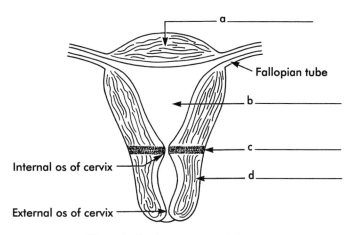

Fig. 4-3. Basic structure of the uterus.

40-41   3. a. _____

              b. _____

              c. _____

              d. _____

The 3 main tissue layers forming the uterine wall moving from the exterior to the interior are:

              e. _myometrium_____

              f. _endometrium_____

              g. _perimetrium_____

The baby must be able to travel through the bony pelvic passageway if he or she is to be born normally. Identify the bones, joints, and landmarks indicated in the following three drawings of the pelvis.

Fig. 4-4. The pelvis, anterior view

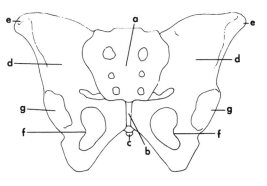

46   4. a. _____   e. _____

              b. _____   f. _____

              c. _____   g. _____

              d. _____

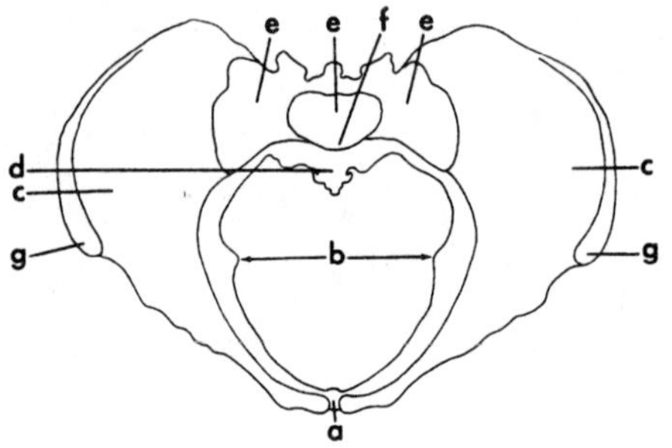

Fig. 4-5. The pelvic inlet.

47

5. a. _____   e. _____

    b. _____   f. _____

    c. _____   g. _____

    d. _____

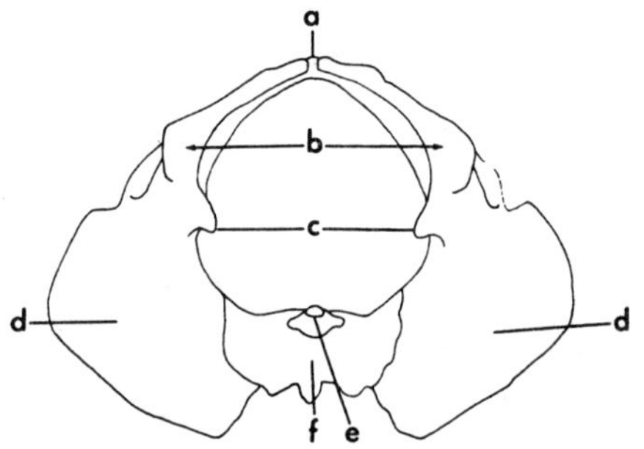

Fig. 4-6. The pelvic outlet.

47

6. a. _____   e. _____

    b. _____   f. _____

    c. _____   g. _____

    d. _____

47

7. On Figs. 4-5 and 4-6 trace the inlet (iliopectineal line) and the outlet with a pencil.

49

8. List four possible causes of distorted pelvic canals.

    a. _____

    b. _____

    c. _____

    d. _____

52

9. Even in the absence of any history of the causes of the distortion listed in question 8, the evaluation of pelvic adequacy still can be of special importance. What are three other instances when a knowledge of the size and shape of the pelvis or its contents is critical? Presence of:

    a. _____

    b. _____

    c. _____

49-52

10. List four ways that pelvic size, contour, and contents can be evaluated.

    a. _pelvimetry._

    b. _Internal palpition_

    c. _External palpition_

    d. _ultrasonogram._

11. Using Fig. 4-7, draw in the diagonal and obstetric conjugates that are estimates of anteroposterior pelvic size.

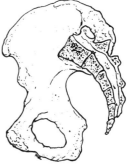

Fig. 4-7. Female pelvis, sagittal section.

47, 50

12. Using Fig. 4-6, draw in the most important transverse diameter of the outlet that can be measured externally.

50

13. It is important that the obstetrical patient have an opportunity to empty her bladder just before a pelvic examination. This preparation makes the internal measurements of the diagonal conjugate (CD) easier. To determine the CD, the physician tries to reach the:
    a. Inner superior border of the pubis
    b. Distance between the ischial spines
    c. Sacral promontory
    d. Coccyx

50

14. The shortest pelvic anteroposterior diameter of the inlet we can clinically estimate is the:
    a. True conjugate
    b. Obstetric conjugate
    c. Diagonal conjugate
    d. Interspinous diameter

50

15. The distance between the ischial tuberosities (TI) helps to indicate the space available to the infant:
    a. To enter the true pelvis
    b. To rotate within the pelvis
    c. To exit the true pelvis

46

16. The progressive differences in the diameter and shape of the bony pelvic canal are largely responsible for the changes in position of the infant's head during labor. These changes are called:
    a. Fetal revolution
    b. Cephalic molding
    c. Internal rotation
    d. External rotation

38

17. Located in the tissue on each side of the vaginal entrance are two glands that produce a mucoid substance. They are:
    a. Bartholin's glands
    b. Skene's glands
    c. Cowper's glands
    d. The bulbourethral glands

43

18. The main muscular supports of the female pelvic contents are:
    a. Levator ani muscles
    b. Gluteus muscles
    c. Round ligaments
    d. Bulbocavernosus muscles

39

19. The *true* perineum of the female is the area of the body that is most likely to tear
during childbirth. To protect it from uncontrolled laceration an episiotomy may be
performed. The true perineum is located:
    a. Just above the vaginal opening
    b. In the area above the vestibule
    c. Between the vagina and the rectum
    d. In the area of the frenulum

41

20. The pelvic adnexa refer to the:
    a. Uterus and ovaries
    b. Bladder and rectum
    c. Ovaries and oviducts
    d. Ovaries

42

21. The muscular contractions of the uterus are:
    a. Under voluntary control
    b. Initiated by motor nerves
    c. Under hormonal control
    d. Initiated by sensory nerves

42

22. Painful sensations that can accompany contractions of the uterus and dilation of
the cervix during labor and childbirth are transmitted by the:
    a. Sympathetic nerve fibers passing through the sixth and seventh thoracic spinal
       nerves
    b. Sympathetic nerve fibers passing through the tenth, eleventh, and twelfth
       thoracic spinal nerves
    c. Sympathetic nerve fibers passing through the vagus nerve complex
    d. Parasympathetic nerve fibers of the vagus nerve complex

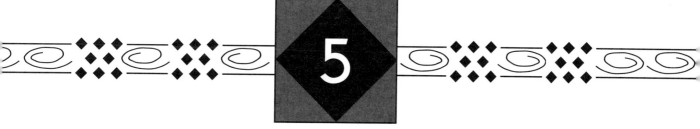

Menstrual Cycle

Page Reference

55-57

1. Human reproduction includes the cyclic preparation for procreation known as the menstrual cycle. This cycle is regulated by hormonal controls produced primarily by two organs, classified as endocrine glands.

   a. These organs are the ____pituitary____ and the ____ovaries____ .

   b. Write the names of the glands, and indicate the hormones manufactured by each gland and their effects.

Endocrine gland	Hormone	Action
Pituitary gland	estrogen	
	progesteron	
Ovary	L H	
	FSH	

55-57

2. Arrange the six different phases of the menstrual cycle in their sequential order according to the tissue they affect:
   Two involving the ovarian cycle:

   a. ____Luteal____   b. ____follicular____

57-58
Four involving the endometrial cycle:

c. _Menstruation_   d. _Proliferative_

e. _Secretory phase_   f. _Ischemic_

3. Define the following terms.

54 a. Menarche _1st period_

60 b. Menorrhagia _heavy m._

60 c. Metrorrhagia _____

55 d. Ovulation _Expulsion of the egg from ovary._

54 e. Menses _menstruation_

60 f. Amenorrhea _____

59 g. Dysmenorrhea _____

54 4. Three structural body changes that occur in young girls as they approach woman-hood are:

a. _hips begins to widen_

b. _delevopment of breast_

c. _fat deposit on buttocks_

58-59, 68 5. Knowledge of different signs of ovulation can be used in treating infertility and implementing family planning. Ovulation usually can be detected by observation of changes in the basal body temperature. Study the basal temperature record in Fig. 5-1 and circle the time of probable ovulation.

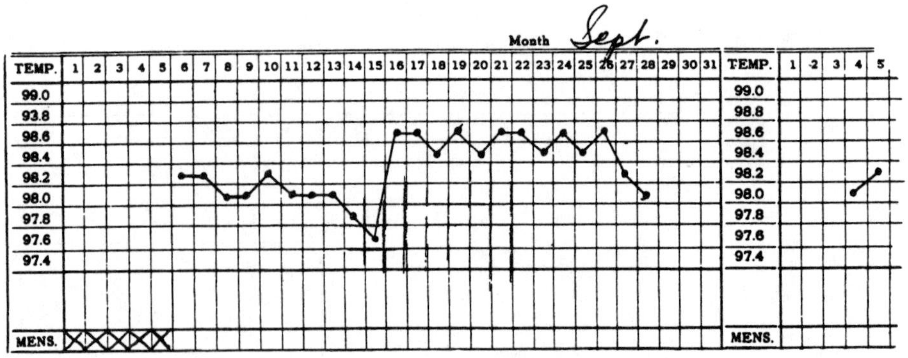

Fig. 5-1. Basal temperature record

59   6. List three ways to prevent or treat premenstrual syndrome (PMS).

        a. _diet — sodium restriction_

        b. _excerises_

        c. _medication — diuretics — edema_

55   7. Menstruation normally occurs at intervals among women of childbearing age. In most women, it appears every:
    a. 14 days for 3 days
    b. 20 days for 5 days
    c. 25 days for 4 days
    d. 28 days for 5 days

54   8. In the United States, the average age that menstruation begins is:
    a. 10 years
    b. 12.5 years
    c. 14 years
    d. 16.5 years

59   9. The most common menstrual disturbance is:
    a. Amenorrhea
    b. Metrorrhagia
    c. Dysmenorrhea
    d. Menorrhagia

59   10. Painful menstruation can accompany all but which one of the following:
    a. Endometrial colonization
    b. Adhesion formation
    c. Prostaglandin production
    d. Ovulation inhibition

55   11. Prostaglandins represent a special group of fatty acids that have far-reaching effects in the body. They are produced:
    a. Only by females
    b. Only by males
    c. By many organs of the body
    d. Only by the endometrium

59   12. Treatment of primary dysmenorrhea may include all of the following *EXCEPT*:
    a. Medication: aspirin, ibuprofen, naproxen
    b. Oral contraceptives: reducing endometrium
    c. Heat, rest, exercise, sodium reduction
    d. Surgery: hymenectomy, uterine repositioning

57   13. When an ovum within a graafian follicle matures and is expelled from the ovary, the follicle becomes what is called the:
    a. Fertility index
    b. Follicular residual
    c. Ovarian residue
    d. Corpus luteum

55   14. Ovulation is sometimes associated with fleeting lower abdominal pain called:
                 a. Mittelschmerz
                 b. Colic
                 c. Peritonitis
                 d. Ileus

58   15. When cervical mucus is profuse and thin (a quality called spinnbarkeit):
                 a. Entry by sperm into the cervix is enhanced
                 b. There is less possibility of pregnancy occurring
                 c. Menstruation will occur within 5 days
                 d. "Ferning" disappears under the influence of estrogen

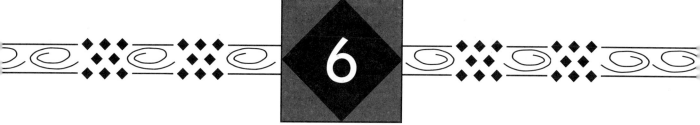

Male Reproduction System

Page Reference

1. Although the paternal role in physical reproduction is relatively brief, it is no less worthy of study than the maternal role. Identify all the lettered anatomic areas of the male reproductive system in Fig. 6-1, and describe the function of the anatomy indicated by the boldface letters and asterisks.

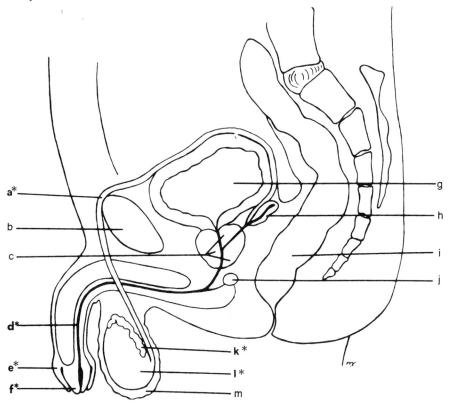

Fig. 6-1. Male pelvic anatomy and reproductive system, sagittal section.

31

65   a.* _____

62, 64   b. _____

63-64   c. _____

62, 63   d.* _____

62   e.* _____

62   f.* _____

64   g. _____

64-65   h. _____

64   i. _____

63-65   j. _____

65   k.* _____

63, 65   l.* _____

63   m. _____

62   2. Puberty or _____maturation_____

occurs on the average at ___14___ years in the male. Male puberty involves: (list four different aspects)

_____Semen production_____

_____deepening voice_____

_____facial hair_____

_____wet dreams_____

64   3. The testis in the male corresponds to the following structure in the female:
           a. Uterus
           b. Ovary
           c. Fallopian tubes
           d. Bartholin's gland

63   4. All of the following regarding scrotal and testicular positions are correct *EXCEPT*:
           a. The left side of the scrotum is often lower than the right
           b. If cold, the testes are moved closer to the body
           c. If warm, the testes are moved away from the body
           d. High scrotal temperatures encourage sperm production

64

5. Testicular cancer, the leading cause of death in young men aged 15-35, is associated with all of the following *EXCEPT*:
   a. Undescended testicle
   b. Underweight
   c. Female relations with breast cancer
   d. Family history

65

6. Three paired glands add secretions to the spermatozoa to influence the sperm's motility and life span. They are:
   a. Vas deferens, seminal vesicle, and prostate
   b. Prostate, seminal vesicle, and ejaculatory duct
   c. Seminal vesicle, prostate, and bulbourethral gland
   d. Cowper's gland, Skene's gland, and prostate

64

7. In women, female characteristics are stimulated by estrogen. In the male, masculine characteristics are stimulated by:
   a. Testosterone
   b. FSH
   c. ICSH
   d. LH

65

8. Male sex cells mature within the:
   a. Seminal vesicles
   b. Epididymides   — Stored in seminal vesicles
   c. Spermatic cords
   d. Bulbourethral glands

Fertility Management

Page Reference

66

1. List five components of a comprehensive family planning program that seeks to manage fertility by a variety of methods.

_____

_____

_____

_____

_____

66

2. Indicate six areas of philosophic difference that may cause various individuals or groups to endorse, tolerate, or condemn certain methods of family planning.

67

3. The three approaches designed to prevent intrauterine growth of a fetus while permitting sexual intercourse are those that control:

   a. _____

   b. _____

   c. _____

67-72   4. List five methods of preventing fertilization and the advantages and disadvantages
              of each.

Table 7-1. Contraceptive methods preventing fertilization

Contraceptive technique	Advantages	Disadvantages	Failure rate (typical use)	STD/HIV protection

72-73   5. List three methods of preventing ovulation and the advantages and disadvantages of each.

Table 7-2. Contraceptive methods preventing ovulation

Technique	Advantages	Disadvantages	STD/HIV protection

72   6. List three possible side effects of oral contraceptives (OCs).

a. _____

b. _____

c. _____

72

7. Indicate three important possible complications of OCs, particularly combination forms:

   a. _____

   b. _____

   c. _____

67-68

8. What is meant by Natural Family Planning (NFP) and how does it differ from the Fertility Awareness Method (FAM)?

74

9. The subject of abortion remains highly controversial and emotionally charged. What was the 1973 United States Supreme Court decision initiated by *Roe v. Wade* regarding abortion? (List three aspects.)

   a. _____

   _____

   _____

   b. _____

   _____

   _____

   c. _____

   _____

   _____

74   10. How may the 1989 Supreme Court decision regarding *Webster v. Reproductive Health Services* affect abortion availability?

76   11. List four surgical interventions used to limit childbearing through sterilization.

      a. _lia   tubal   ligatwon_____

      b. _Band and_____

      c. _Vaginal tubal sterlizatin_____

      d. _____

76-77   12. Fertility in human terms can be defined as "the ability of the body to reproduce." Infertility is technically defined as:

      _____

      _____

      _____

77   13. In an attempt to determine the cause of a couple's infertility, the man is evaluated first, because either partner may have reproductive problems and investigation of the man is less difficult. List three tests or examinations that may be performed in addition to a complete history and physical examination to evaluate the man's reproductive capacity.

      a. _norman   analisis_____

      b. _X - Ray studies_____

      c. _Testicular   biopsy_____

77   14. List four methods that can be used in addition to a complete history and physical examination to evaluate the woman's reproductive capacity.

a. Basal body temperature

b. L H levels in urine

c. Biopsy of endometrium

d. VIScosity of cervical mucus

67   15. One of the national health objectives for year 2000 is the reduction of unwanted or earlier than planned pregnancies to:
a. 10% of all pregnancies
b. 20% of all pregnancies
c. 30% of all pregnancies
d. 40% of all pregnancies

74   16. The reliability of many forms of contraception depends on the understanding and conscientious technique of the user. However, one kind of contraceptive device that does not depend on this aspect for a 98% to 99.2% rate of effectiveness is the:
a. Pill
b. Condom
c. Diaphragm
d. IUD

73   17. Controversy exists regarding how IUDs control pregnancy, but it is believed that:
a. Fertilization does not occur
b. Ovulation does not take place
c. Implantation is not completed

74   18. Complications diagnosed infrequently with IUDs but worth consideration include the following. Which occurrence is most common?
a. Uterine infection
b. Uterine perforation
c. Uterine cramping and bleeding
d. Spontaneous expulsion

74   19. Although IUDs are thought not to be the cause, users who become pregnant have been found to experience an increased incidence of:
a. Male infants
b. Ectopic pregnancies
c. Twinning
d. Placenta previa

72   20. One of the reasons a douche is not considered a method of contraception is that:
a. Sperm may enter the cervix as rapidly as 10 to 90 seconds after ejaculation
b. The technique may cause infection
c. It does not alter the vaginal pH
d. It usually is performed improperly

73
21. Women who take oral contraceptives are known to have an increased risk of thrombus and embolus formation if they:
   a. Are over 35 years of age and smoke
   b. Have poor diets
   c. Drink alcohol
   d. Take narcotics

77
22. Hormonal stimulation with menotropins (Pergonal) has become a source of special interest because of the increased possibility of:
   a. Multiple pregnancies
   b. Maternal morbidity
   c. Gross congenital malformations
   d. Heightened infant intelligence

1. Premenstrual tension syndrome has been variously defined, explained, and blamed for numerous female symptoms and behaviors. What concepts are currently advanced involving this puzzling phenomenon? What types of management have been recommended and what impact does the syndrome have on family function?

REFERENCES

Cortese J and Brown MA: Coping responses of men whose partners experience premenstrual symptomatology, J Obstet Gynecol Neonatal Nurs (JOGNN)
18(5):405-412, 1989.

Hsia LSY and Long MH: Premenstrual syndrome, J Nurse Midwifery 35(6):351-7, 1990.

Lindow KB: Premenstrual syndrome: family impact and nursing implications, JOGNN 20(2) 135-8, 1991.

Mitchell ES: The elusive premenstrual syndrome, NAACOG Clin Issues Perinatal Women's Health Nurs 2(3):294-303, 1991.

Ornitz AW and Brown MA: Family coping and premenstrual symptomatology, JOGNN 22(1):49-55, 1993.

2. The perfect contraceptive method is yet to be found. Discuss some of the problems raised in three of the following references.

REFERENCES

Engel NS: Update on cancer risk and oral contraceptives, MCN 15(1):37, 1990.

Fehring RJ: New technology in natural family planning, JOGNN 20(3):199-205, 1991.

Franklin D: The birth control bind, Health 6(4):42-52, 1992.

Kaunitz AM: DMPA: New contraceptive option, Contemp OB/GYN 38(1):19-34, 1993.

King J: Helping patients choose an appropriate method of birth control MCV 17(2):91-95, 1992.

Lethbridge D: Coitus interruptus as a method of birth control, JOGNN 20(1):80-85, 1991.

Lommel L and Taylor D: Adolescent use of contraceptives NAACOG Clin Issues Perinatal Women's Health Nurs 3(2):199-208, 1992.

Low M: Personal values and contraceptive choices, NAACOG Clin Issues Perinatal Women's Health Nurs 3(2):192-198, 1992.

Nurses' Association of the American College of Obstetricians and Gynecologists: Contraceptive options: OGN nursing practice resource, Washington DC, 1991, NAACOG.

Pollack A: Long-term consequences of female and male sterilization, Contemp OB/GYN 38(8):41-54, 1993.

Runner J: If you're asked about Norplant, RN 55(6):44-47, 1992.

Runner J: Women's health—Depo Provera: a "new" contraceptive option and RU-486: an option thus far denied, 1994 medical and health annual, Chicago, 1993, Encyclopedia Britannica Inc.

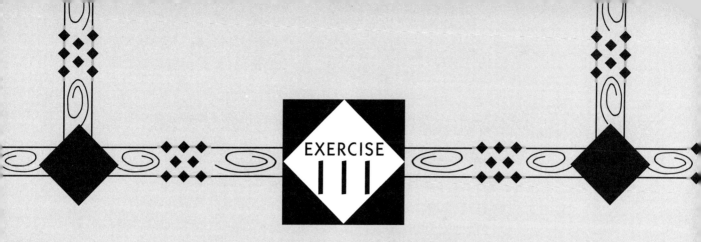

PREGNANCY

Waiting is almost always difficult, and the lengthy period of silent fetal growth within the uterus represents a waiting period of special concern and wonder for the mother and father expecting the birth of a child. This prenatal experience is of special significance in helping to determine the physical, social, and psychological readiness of the parents and the basic physical and intellectual capabilities of the developing young individual. The interval of gestation usually is filled with mixed emotions, which include uncertainty, fantasy, frustration, anger, annoyance, anxiety, excitement, pride, and hope. Nurses in the office, clinic, or hospital play an important role as they seek to promote health, prevent abnormality, or help treat disease on behalf of the pregnant woman, her unborn child, and the family.

CLINICAL TIE-IN

1. Talk to a friend or relative who is a new mother. Have her share some of the things she found difficult during her pregnancy. Could nurses be of any assistance in solving or reducing these problems? Would the physician, nutritionist, social worker, clergy, or psychiatrist help meet the needs expressed?

2. If you are assigned to participate in a prenatal clinic as part of your clinical experience, determine the following:
   a. What types of patients are eligible to attend?
   b. How are the expenses of the clinic met?
   c. How do patients get to the clinic?
   d. How long do most of the patients wait before their appointments are completed?
   e. Are there any babysitting facilities?
   f. Are there any attempts to teach health concepts to groups of patients at the clinic? Approximately how much time is spent by the nurses or physicians teaching the patients on an individual basis?
   g. Do the nurses seem to know the patients who have come several times? Do they express interest and concern for the individual patient?
   h. Are there any linguistic or cultural barriers between the patients and staff?

3. Read the prenatal records of patients who recently have been or soon will be admitted for delivery. What problems were identified, and how were they handled?

4. What kinds of premarital or prenatal tests or examinations are required by law in your state?

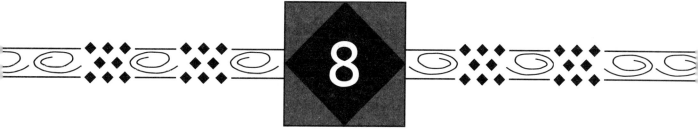

Conception and Fetal Development

Page Reference

83   1. Define the following terms.

a. Conception (fertilization) _____

_____

_____

85   b. Zygote _____

_____

_____

84-85   c. Morula _____

_____

_____

84-85   d. Blastocyst _____

_____

_____

84   e. Chorionic villi _____

_____

_____

45

84   f. Chorion _____

_____

_____

84   g. Amnion _____

_____

_____

84, 86   h. Yolk sac _____

_____

_____

84, 86   i. Embryonic disc _____

_____

_____

86, 88 + Glossary   j. Embryo _____

_____

_____

94 + Glossary   k. Fetus _____

_____

_____

84, 93 + Glossary   l. Placenta _____

_____

_____

93   2. List five functions of the placenta.

a. _____

b. _____

c. _____

d. _____

e. _____

94   3. Match the stage of fetal maturation with the prenatal calendar. (Letters can be used more than once.)

   ____ About 7 1/2 inches, 3 1/3 oz

   ____ Calcified skeleton begun

   ____ Fetal heart tone heard by
         nonultrasonic fetoscope

   ____ Sex visible

   ____ Fetus

   a.   End of 8 weeks
   b.   End of 12 weeks
   c.   End of 16 weeks
   d.   18-20 weeks

95   4. Label the key structures (a-f) indicated in the flow of the fetal circulation pictured in Fig. 8-1. Describe on the next page each structure's function and what normally happens to each structure after birth or by 2 or 3 weeks.

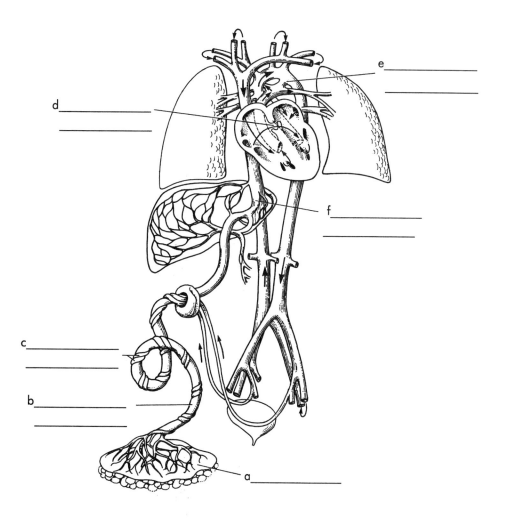

Fig. 8-1. Fetal circulation

Key structures	Fetal function	Destiny following birth of infant
g. Placenta	_____	_____
	_____	_____
h. Umbilical vein	_____	_____
	_____	_____
i. Umbilical arteries	_____	_____
	_____	_____
j. Foramen ovale	_____	_____
	_____	_____
k. Ductus arteriosus	_____	_____
	_____	_____
l. Ductus venosus	_____	_____
	_____	_____

98, Table 8-2

5. Measures of fetal assessment.
   a. List four determinations or techniques that may help discover an unborn infant's age or growth:

   (1.) _____

   (2.) _____

   (3.) _____

   (4.) _____

   b. What type of specimen is often analyzed to help determine an infant's

   respiratory maturity?_____

   c. List eight ways that may assist in evaluating an infant's well-being.

   (1.) _____

   (2.) _____

   (3.) _____

   (4.) _____

   (5.)_____

(6.) _____

(7.) _____

(8.) _____

101-105   6. The signs and symptoms of pregnancy may be divided into three classifications according to their reliability. Note presumptive indications with ??, probable with +?, and positive with ++.

    _____ a. Urinary frequency

    _____ b. Abdominal striae

    _____ c. Fetal heart tone

    _____ d. Fetal movement felt by a trained examiner

    _____ e. Positive pregnancy test

    _____ f. Nausea and vomiting

    _____ g. Elevation of basal body temperature

    _____ h. Hegar's sign

    _____ i. Chadwick's sign

    _____ j. Fetal skeleton detected by ultrasound or x-ray examination

84   7. The term "gestational age" (GA) refers to the length of a human pregnancy calculated from the:
a. Date of ovulation
b. Date of conception
c. First day of last menses
d. Last day of last menses

84   8. The duration of a normal gestation using menstrual age is:
a. 36 weeks
b. 38 weeks
c. 40 weeks
d. 42 weeks

84   9. The sex of an infant will be female if she receives from her father:
a. One X chromosome
b. One Y chromosome
c. One Y and one X chromosome
d. 23 chromosomes

84, 104   10. Present pregnancy tests are based on the fact that chorionic villi secrete:
a. FSH
b. LH
c. hCG
d. ICSH

84

11. When pregnancy occurs, the inner layer of the uterus or endometrium becomes known as the:
    a. Amnion
    b. Chorion
    c. Ectoderm
    d. Decidua

84

12. The process by which a fertilized ovum embeds into the uterine wall is called:
    a. Fertilization
    b. Implantation
    c. Ovulation
    d. Migration

84

13. The intact "bag of waters" or membranes containing amniotic fluid helps protect the fetus from all of the following EXCEPT:
    a. Infection
    b. Temperature change
    c. Trauma
    d. Asphyxia

84, 99

14. The process of extracting a fluid sample from the "bag of waters" is called:
    a. Thoracentesis
    b. Amniocentesis
    c. Paracentesis
    d. Culdocentesis

96

15. There are two types of twins. All the statements below regarding fraternal twins are true EXCEPT:
    a. They occur less frequently
    b. They develop from 2 ova
    c. They each have a placenta
    d. They each have an amniotic sac

96

16. Drugs or conditions that produce fetal structural defects are termed:
    a. Teratogens
    b. Androgens
    c. Estrogens
    d. Hallucinogens

103-104

17. The fundus or top of the uterus usually is palpated about halfway between the maternal umbilicus and pubic bone at:
    a. 12 weeks
    b. 16 weeks
    c. 20 weeks
    d. 24 weeks

102

18. The violet coloration of the vagina, cervix, and vulva, which usually is considered a presumptive sign of pregnancy, is known as:
    a. Hegar's sign
    b. Quickening
    c. Chadwick's sign
    d. Goodell's sign

105   19. Before the twentieth week of development, the fetal heart is best detected:
          a. At the center of the pubic hair line
          b. Halfway between the pubis and umbilicus
          c. In the lower left abdominal quadrant
          d. In the lower right abdominal quadrant

105   20. All of the following are positive signs of pregnancy *EXCEPT*:
          a. Fetal heartbeat
          b. Quickening
          c. Fetal movement
          d. Ultrasound view of fetus

103   21. A woman expecting her first baby usually experiences a sudden relief from short-
          ness of breath about 2 weeks before her delivery. This change is the result of a
          process called:
          a. Quickening
          b. Flexion
          c. Implantation
          d. Lightening

105   22. In maternity nursing, the enduring mutual affection that should develop between
          parents and their infant is often called:
          a. Dependency
          b. Attachment
          c. Symbiosis
          d. Interaction

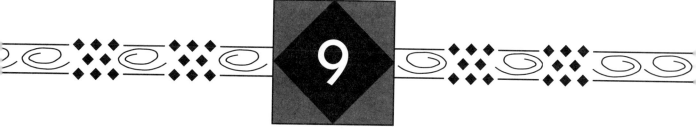

Pregnancy and
Prenatal Care

Page Reference

110   1. Define the following key terms:

a. Viable _____

_____

b. Primigravida _____

_____

c. Primipara (primip) _____

_____

d. Multipara (multip) _____

_____

e. Nullipara _____

_____

The physiology of pregnancy:
The most dramatic changes in the anatomy and physiology of the pregnant women involve her reproductive system. However, these changes affect all other body systems. Identify as indicated *alterations in each of the body systems below* that should influence nursing care.

111   2. Cardiovascular system. (List four)

a. _____

_____

b. _____

_____

c. _____

_____

d. _____

_____

111

3. Gastrointestinal system. (List three)

a. _____

_____

b. _____

_____

c. _____

_____

111-112

4. Urinary system. (List two)

a. _____

_____

b. _____

_____

112

5. Indicate the typical psychological changes of pregnancy by identifying the key word or words that describe the changing emotional outlook of most expectant women during each trimester.

a. _____

b. _____

c. _____

112

6. State the *broad objectives* of prenatal care as formulated by the U.S. Department of Health and Human Services in 1989.

_____

_____

_____

115 7. In order to achieve the systematic examination, observation, and anticipatory guidance desired, prenatal care is comprised of three main components. They are:

a. _____

_____

_____

b. _____

_____

_____

c. _____

_____

_____

115 8. A National Health Objective for the United States by the year 2000 involving prenatal care is:

_____

_____

_____

116 9. Identify the four main types of information that usually are obtained as a result of the initial prenatal pelvic examination.

a. _____

_____

b. _____

_____

c. _____

_____

d. _____

_____

117-118

10. List six laboratory tests that are ordered frequently in a busy maternity center to help evaluate the status of an expectant mother.

a. _____

_____

b. _____

_____

c. _____

_____

d. _____

_____

e. _____

_____

f. _____

_____

118

11. Expectant mothers are cautioned to report certain signs or symptoms when they occur. List nine such danger signs.

a. _____

b. _____

c. _____

d. _____

e. _____

f. _____

g. _____

h. _____

i. _____

12. Prenatal visits to an appropriate health care provider should continue periodically throughout pregnancy. Each of the following statements should be marked true or false by circling the response. If you mark a statement false, you must alter the statement to make it form a relevant, correct sentence. Do not correct the sentence by simply making it negative.

118   T (F)   a. During the first 28 weeks of pregnancy, most women are asked to visit their health care provider every 6 weeks.

_____ *g u weeks a/er* _____

_____

_____

118   T (F)   b. Routinely, each visit will include weight, TPR, B/P measurements; (a pelvic examination tests for hemoglobin levels and urine glucose and albumin.) *not*

done Routinely

_____

_____

117   (T) F   c. Only 4% of all babies whose birth dates were determined using Nagele's rule arrive on that day, but all born within 2 weeks of the calculated EDD are considered full term.

_____

_____

_____

117   T F   d. Rh <u>positive</u> mothers need special supervision, which includes increasingly frequent antibody titers and an injection of Rho GAM at about 28 weeks.

Rh negative _____

_____

_____

119   (T) F   e. A blood glucose test may be ordered at 24-28 weeks because during pregnancy urine glucose is not diagnostic for diabetes.

_____

_____

_____

118   T (F)   f. Gradual increasing fetal movement, and retarded growth in uterine size and fundal height are all signs of possible infant jeopardy.

decrease in

_____

_____

_____

115   13. Joan Wonder is a nicely groomed 42 year old nervously visiting her obstetrician after an 11 year interval—the age of her youngest and fourth child. Could it be that she is pregnant? Later, using the G/TPAL code, Dr. Holmes notes on her

record 5/3013. Is she pregnant? _____
How is the code interpreted?

_____

_____

_____

_____

_____

116   14. Leslie Little is a lively 19 year old. Both she and her husband Don are excited about the possibility of having a baby son or daughter. She finds it difficult to sit calmly as she anticipates her first prenatal visit. She has walked to the drinking fountain twice in the last 40 minutes. What courtesy should be extended to Leslie and all patients before their examination? Why?

_____

_____

_____

15. Fill in the table for nutrients most often deficient in diets that could be supplied by a balanced diet.

	Nutrient	Role in body/baby building and maintenance	Deficiency (D)/ Excess (E) Problems	Sources
121-122	Vitamin B_6 Pyridoxine			
123	Vitamin D			
121	Vitamin E			
122	Folate Folacin (Folic acid)			
122-123	Calcium			
123	Zinc			
123	Magnesium			

122

16. Iron deficiency anemia is the most common anemia of pregnancy.

It is associated with (a.) _____ ,

(b.) _____, (c.) _____. Iron

is necessary to manufacture (d.)_____ in
both maternal and fetal blood cells.

17. The RDA for iron doubles to 30 mg during pregnancy and is difficult to achieve by diet alone. The Institute of Medicine recommends the supplementation of

(a.) _____ of ferrous iron per day beginning at approxi-

mately (b.) _____ gestation. Identify two sources rich in

iron: (c.) _____ (d.) _____ .

18. Current weight gain recommendations are commonly based on prepregnancy weight for height. A normal weight woman should gain approximately

_____ pounds.

19. Prepare an analysis of your diet of yesterday (or that of a woman you know). If yesterday's food intake was not typical, select one day that was more representative. A sample 24 hour dietary recall or "food diary" and completed and blank Daily Food Analysis sheets may be found in the Answer Section of this Study Guide to serve as a pattern for your analysis. The instructions below should also be of assistance.
   a. Write your food diary on a separate sheet of note paper, listing everything you ate chronologically during the 24 hour period. Your food intake analysis will be based not on a calorie count, but on the number of servings consumed from the seven food groups displayed in the Daily Food Guide on page 125 in the text.
      (1.) List all foods eaten including the contents of mixtures such as sandwiches, casseroles, and salads.
      (2.) Include jelly, butter, sugar and milk in coffee etc. Water and unadorned coffee and tea are not officially part of this analysis, but you may want to note the amount of such intake. Plain water is better than coffee or tea both of which contain diuretics. Most references recommend 6 to 8 cups of water daily.
      (3.) Estimate amounts consumed as accurately as possible.
   b. Use the Daily Food Guide and Daily Food Analysis with the food diary you prepared. Consult the "One Serving Equals" section of the Guide. Determine and record how many servings of what Food Groups you ate.
   c. Identify the number of servings of each Food Group needed by a nonpregnant (NP) woman. Be aware that you must choose 2 requirements based on age for this category. You must fill in those blanks on the Food Analysis form. (Food Groups #2 and #3).
   d. Add up the number of servings you consumed in each Food Group. Calculate the differences between your needs according to this Guide and what you actually ate. Write your + or - calculations in the Differences column.

e. Think of and record an item you could increase or add to your diet to supply any deficit discovered. If your serving totals are excessive, what could be deleted? Excessive counts are not usually detrimental unless items used contain a predominance of empty calories. See note at the bottom of the Daily Food Guide.

f. Indicate how the intake recorded would need to be changed if the woman whose diet was just analyzed became pregnant. Fill in changes based on the different requirements of pregnancy (P) stated in the Guide and complete the summary below.

	Diet Evaluation Summary			
Group	**Record of Intake for One Day**		**Modifications Needed to Meet Requirements Recommended**	
		Servings	**Nonpregnant**	**Pregnant/Lactating**
1				
2				
3				
4				
5				
6				
7				

128

20. Discuss general exercise for healthy women with uncomplicated pregnancies.
   a. What benefits does regular exercise offer? (List three)

   _____

   _____

   _____

   b. Identify four sports or types of exercise or exercise conditions that are not recommended for mothers-to-be.

   _____

   _____

   _____

   _____

   c. After the fourth month, expectant mothers should not exercise in the supine position. Why?

   _____

   _____

   _____

   _____

   d. The American College of Obstetricians and Gynecologists have recommended that exercising expectant mothers should: (List three considerations)

   _____

   _____

   _____

   e. What are Kegal exercises and how may they benefit the prenatal woman or any woman? (Define and list four ways)

   _____

   _____

   _____

   _____

   _____

129-131   21. Briefly state the frequently recommended methods of prevention and treatment for the following common discomforts of pregnancy.

a. Mild to moderate nausea and vomiting

_____

_____

_____

_____

_____

130-131   b. Heartburn

_____

_____

_____

_____

_____

132   c. Constipation

_____

_____

_____

_____

_____

132   d. Varicosities of the legs

_____

_____

_____

_____

_____

133   e. *Trichomonas vaginalis* infection

_____

_____

_____

_____

_____

134   f. *Candida albicans* infection

_____

_____

_____

_____

135   22. Community Education Resources for Childbirth: Over the years since the first edition of *Childbirth Without Fear* was written, many different courses have been formed to share beneficial information and supportive techniques to be used during pregnancy, childbirth and parenthood.
               a Briefly state the main psychoprophylactic principle taught by French obstetrician Fernand Lamaze:

_____

_____

_____

               b. Explain how this is applied during labor and birth:

_____

_____

_____

_____

134   23. Identify four different sponsors of classes designed to help expectant parents prepare for the changes in their lives:

_____

_____

_____

_____

_____

117   24. Using Nagele's rule, if a pregnant woman's last normal menstrual period occurred between December 10 and December 15, 1993, what would be her calculated due date?
a. September 10, 1994
b. September 17, 1994
c. September 3, 1994
d. September 22, 1994

120   25. It is recommended that a normal healthy pregnant woman of any age consume as part of her daily diet particularly after her first trimester, an additional:
a. 200 calories
b. 300 calories
c. 400 calories
d. 500 calories

124, 126   26. Using current literature, a woman who is 5 feet 6 inches tall, who weighs 163 lbs at the start of her pregnancy, generally would be advised to gain:
a. 28-40 lbs
b. 25-35 lbs
c. 15-25 lbs
d. 15 lbs

125   27. Two excellent sources of vitamin C are:
a. Broccoli, strawberries
b. Sweet potatoes, oranges
c. Pumpkin, raw cabbage
d. Apricots, yams

121   28. A diet depending only on animal sources of protein is likely to:
a. Be less costly
b. Involve incomplete proteins
c. Contain more cholesterol
d. Contain less fat

111   29. Hemoglobin and hematocrit levels that usually signal the presence of anemia in a pregnant woman are:
a. Hemoglobin less than 11 g/dl, hematocrit less than 33%
b. Hemoglobin less than 12 g/dl, hematocrit less than 36%
c. Hemoglobin less than 13 g/dl, hematocrit less than 39%
d. Hemoglobin less than 14 g/dl, hematocrit less than 42%

124-126   30. Pregnant women sometimes desire to eat unusual or strange combinations of foods. The desire to eat nonfood substances such as laundry starch or clay may interfere with good nutrition. This practice is called:
a. Mining
b. Lightening
c. Argo
d. Pica

126   31. Expectant mothers are routinely examined for signs of pregnancy-induced-hyper-
tension (PIH), a leading cause of maternal mortality. In addition to hypertension,
what other signs of this disease could be identified during the prenatal period.
   a. Edema of face or hands; glycosuria
   b. Edema of face or hands; albuminuria
   c. Infection, excessive weight gain
   d. Blurred vision, glycosuria

124   32. After the first trimester of pregnancy, it is usually recommended that a pregnant
woman gain about:
   a. 1/4 pound per week
   b. 1/2 pound per week
   c. 1 pound per week
   d. 2 or 3 pounds per week

129   33. The best time for a pregnant woman to travel is during:
   a. The first trimester of pregnancy
   b. The second trimester of pregnancy
   c. The third trimester of pregnancy
   d. The eighth month of pregnancy

129   34. To promote her comfort and safety as pregnancy progresses, a woman's wardrobe
usually needs some changes. All of the following probably would be beneficial
EXCEPT:
   a. A larger bra size
   b. Lower heeled shoes
   c. Elastic-topped hose
   d. Light, comfortable clothes

133   35. For immediate relief of leg cramps, one helpful action is:
   a. Pointing your toe while stretching
   b. Applying cold compresses to the calf muscle
   c. Taking calcium supplements immediately
   d. Pushing down in knee; pulling foot toward knee

133   36. Even when not pregnant, women should not douche for all the reasons below
EXCEPT:
   a. Douching may initiate uterine contraction
   b. Douching may force bacteria into the uterus
   c. Douching may cause an air embolism
   d. Douching may wash away normal flora

136   37. Among these baby shower gifts, which should not be used with an infant?
   a. A small pillow
   b. Cotton diapers
   c. Stretch cotton shirts
   d. Plastic diaper covers

137   38. The concepts of Yin and Yang often followed in Asiatic cultures have similarities to
the hot-cold theory of disease and health encountered especially in the:
   a. African-American culture
   b. Hispanic culture
   c. Arabic culture
   d. Alaskan lifestyle

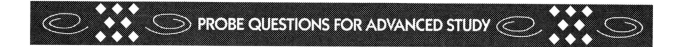

PROBE QUESTIONS FOR ADVANCED STUDY

1. The unborn child is the recipient of many maternal influences that impact the developing infant. Usually, these influences are benign or beneficial; occasionally they may be terrible and teratogenic. Describe three prenatal poisons, the fetal damage they can cause, and what is being done to stop their use or combat their effects.

REFERENCES

Blume SB, Counts SJ and Turnball JM: When you first suspect substance abuse, Contemp OB/GYN 38(3) 74-94, 1993.

Brown MJ, Bellinger D and Matthews J: In utero lead exposure, MCN 15(2):94-96, 1990.

Byrne MW and Lerner HM: Communicating with addicted women in labor, MCN 17(1):22-26, 1992.

Campinha-Bacote J and Bragg EJ: Chemical assessment in maternity care, MCN 18(1):24-28, 1993.

Dorris M: The broken cord, New York, 1990, Harper Collins. (Winner of 1989 National Book Critics Circle Award-a biography recounting the impact of fetal alcohol syndrome).

Dorris M: The tragedy of fetal alcohol syndrome: a father's reflection, 1994 medical and health annual, Chicago, 1993, Enclopedia Britannica Inc.

International Childbirth Association, Inc.: ICEA position statement: substance abuse during pregnancy, Minneapolis, Minn, Feb 1992.

Jacques JT and Snyder N: Newborn victims of addiction, RN 54(4):47-52, 1991.

McDonald AD, Armstrong BG and Sloan M: Cigarette, alcohol and coffee consumption and abortion; prematurity and congenital defects, Am J Public Health 82(1):85-93, 1992.

McKim EM: Caffeine and its effects on pregnancy and the neonate, J Nurse-Midwifery 36(4):226-231, 1991.

Medoff-Cooper B and Verklan T: Substance abuse, NAACOG Clin Issues Perinatal Women's Health Nurs 3(1):114-128, 1992.

Pletsch PK: Birth defect prevention: nursing interventions, JOGNN 19(6):482-487, 1990.

Reiskin H: Alcohol and other drug education videos, MCN 17(4):210-213, 1992.

Starn J et al: We can encourage pregnant substance abusers to seek prenatal care MCN 18(3):148-152, 1993.

Sweet OR and Bryan P: The working woman's Lamaze handbook, New York, 1992, Hyperion.

2. As we approach the twenty-first century, a number of fairly new technologies are being used that may make possible certain corrective or selective procedures involving the unborn child. What types of procedures have been attempted? How successful have they been? What ethical, legal, or financial problems may they pose?

REFERENCES

Carey B: Chance of a lifetime, Health 8(3):91-98, 1994.

Collins JE: Fetal surgery: changing the outcome before birth, JOGNN 23(2):166-169, 1994.

Goode CJ and Hahn SJ: Oocyte donation and in vitro fertilization: the nurse's role with ethical and legal issues, JOGNN 22(2):106-111, 1993.

Jones SL: Genetic-based and assisted reproductive technology of the 21st century, JOGNN 23(2):160-164, 1994.

Magil B: Fetal surgery: past, present, and future work in this frontier, Contemp OB/GYN 39(1):59-66, 1994.

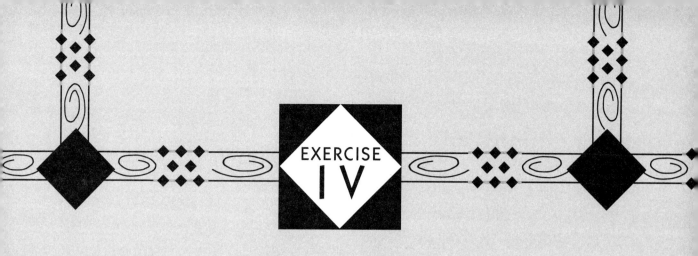

CHILDBIRTH AND POSTPARTUM

The birth of a baby represents both a finale and a commencement. The occasion is filled with expectations, fears, and promised. It makes physical, psychological, and emotional demands on the mother, the baby, and all other members of the family unit. It is a special privilege and a rich educational experience to be present when a baby first enters the extrauterine world and to be part of the health team that seeks to care for the newborn child and his parents. In this exercise, important aspects of the perinatal period are reviewed, and some questions regarding its significance are posed.

CLINICAL TIE-IN

1. Look at the delivery records of your postpartum or newborn patients, or analyze the deliveries you have observed this week. Describe the mechanisms of the passage of the fetus down the birth canal.
2. By what means can the condition of the baby be estimated before he is born? Can you think of three different methods of assessment that were employed with labor patients this week?
3. How many types of obstetrical analgesia have you observed? What effect, if any, have they appeared to have on the mother? On the baby?
4. Compare the first stage of labor (length, dilation patterns, and general tolerance) of three normal primiparas with that of the three normal multiparas of approximately the same age who have received the same type of analgesia or psychoprophylactic preparation. Name three other factors that can influence the course of the first stage of labor.
5. Listen to the conversation of two new mothers. Try to determine what nursing measure or characteristic was most helpful to them during their labors and deliveries and what aspect of nursing care should be improved or reevaluated.
6. Modify the format of pp. 178-180 in text (behavioral expectations and care of the typical labor-delivery patient), and describe the characteristics and nursing care of a mother whom you assisted during labor, comparing and contrasting her experiences with those of the "typical" patient.
7. Today's typical postpartal women and their new babies often have only a few hours of care in a hospital or maternity center setting following their birth experiences. How are their physical, psychological, and educational needs being met? How do the caregivers cope? Who are they? What are some positive aspects of early discharge? What negative situations have been reported? What has been the impact of the federal Family and Medical Leave Act of 1993?
8. Two large and current concerns are the questions involving cost and availability of health care. What financial commitment do various types of childbirth care represent for individuals and families in your community? How much are insurance groups or health plans assisting? Do you have any figures to share?

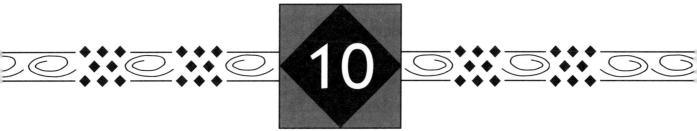

Mechanics of
Labor and Birth

Page Reference

141

1. Indicate the four major factors that determine the progress of labor:

   a. _Passage_

   b. _Passenger_

   c. _Power_

   d. _Psyche_

2. Define the following terms:

142

   a. Presentation _part of the baby comming through the pelvic cannal first_

142, 144

   b. Position _____

142

   c. Attitude _Degree of flexion to the presenting part_

144-145

   d. Station _Relationship of of the presenting part to the ischemial spines of the pelvis_

149

   e. Cervical effacement _____

149-150

   f. Cervical dilation _____

145   3. Using abbreviations, identify the three positions shown in Fig. 10-1

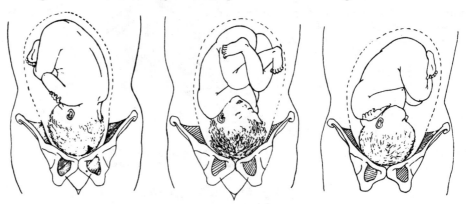

Fig. 10-1. Vertex positions.

a. _____   b. _____

c. _____

147-148   4. Why might a posterior position be associated with a more difficult labor? What problems are encountered? (List two.)

a. _____

b. _____

146   5. Using the abbreviations, identify the three breech types and the three breech positions shown in Fig. 10-2.

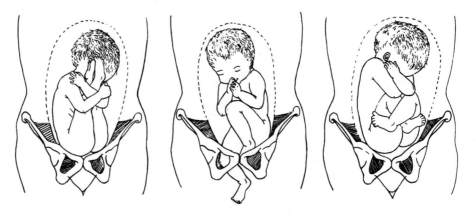

Fig. 10-2. Breech types and positions

a. _____   _____

b. _____   _____

c. _____   _____

150

6. Using the chart below, contrast six characteristics of true and false labor:

True Labor	False Labor

145-146,
148 (Fig. 10-7)

7. List the seven movements that make up the mechanism of labor that the fetus usually follows in the journey to the exterior when the fetus is in the vertex presentation.

a. _____

b. _____

c. _____

d. _____

e. _____

f. _____

g. _____

151-152   8. When labor is not progressing normally, list four options that may be considered by health care providers.

a. _Intensify maternal & fetal monitoring_

b. _Stimulate uterine contraction c̄ oxytocic_

c. _Preparation for c-Section_

d. _Use of sedation for mother_

154   9. List four signs of the separation of the placenta from the uterus:

a. _Increase firmness and rounded shape of pelvis_

b. _Lengthing of umbilical cord from the vagina_

c. _raise ↑ of the uterus to the ambilicus or above_

d. _Sudden appearance of moderate temporary vag. bleeding_

142   10. Most humans enter this world head first. In fact, cephalic presentations occur in:
a. 60% of births
b. 75% of births
c. 85% of births
d. 96% of births

144   11. When a fetus is *LOA, O* stands for:
a. Outer
b. Of
c. Occiput
d. Zero

144   12. Another term for *transverse lie* is:
a. A transverse arrest
b. A shoulder presentation
c. *ROT*
d. A single footling

142   13. An expectant mother's progress in labor may be slowed by the presence of all of the following *EXCEPT*:
a. Her high anxiety levels
b. Her small pelvic dimensions
c. Her baby's vertex presentation
d. Her baby's posterior position

150   14. The first stage of labor ends with the:
a. Appearance of show
b. Rupture of the bag of waters
c. Complete dilation of the cervix
d. Birth of the baby

151   15. The *latent phase* of dilation for a nullipara illustrated by the Friedman Labor Curve
            is considered prolonged if it lasts more than:
            a. 12 hours
            b. 14 hours
            c. 16 hours
            d. 20 hours

151   16. Potentially the most damaging dilation pattern as described by Friedman is:
            a. Prolonged initial effacement
            b. Prolonged latent phase of dilation
            c. Protracted active phase of dilation
            d. Secondary arrest of the maximum slope of dilation

151   17. The Friedman Labor Curve is used to:
            a. Help detect problems of cervical dilation and descent
            b. Identify fetal distress and select proper treatment
            c. Predict length of labor and maternal stress
            d. Assess maternal and fetal tolerance to labor

154   18. The complication of maternal hemorrhage most frequently occurs during the:
            a. First stage of labor
            b. First and second stages of labor
            c. Third stage of labor
            d. Third and fourth stages of labor

154   19. A medication that causes the uterus to contract is called:
            a. An antipyretic
            b. An oxytocic
            c. An antihistamine
            d. A steroid

142   20. Purposeful turning of a fetus from a breech to a cephalic presentation is termed:
            a. External version
            b. Station placement
            c. Precipitous labor
            d. Internal engagement

154   21. A multipara characteristically has a shorter first stage labor than a woman bearing
            her first child. "Multip" first stage labor usually averages:
            a. 4 to 6 hours
            b. 6 to 8 hours
            c. 8 to 10 hours
            d. 10 to 12 hour

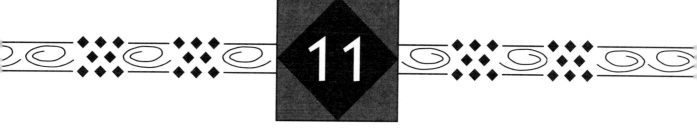

Labor
and Birth

Page Reference

158

1. Within the last 25 years many changes have taken place in the philosophy, content, and delivery of perinatal care. List four consumer demands that have led to the reshaping of maternity care, especially in the period immediately surrounding childbirth.

   a. More natural child birth
   b. more control over birth expenses.
   c. ✓ family participation
   d. lower cost
   e greater access to newborn

Margie Lester, a 24-year-old housewife with an active, normal 2 1/2-year-old son, is at term with her second pregnancy. In preparation for this second, planned baby, she and her husband attended childbirth education classes featuring psychoprophylactic techniques, sponsored by her obstetrician and cooperating hospital maternity department. Her first labor and delivery lasted 20 hours and was complicated by suspected fetal distress, first detected shortly before delivery, manifested by intermittent dips in the fetal heart rate. The baby was quickly delivered vaginally with the assistance of forceps. Apgar scores of 6 and 7 were recorded at 1 and 5 minutes after delivery, and oxygen was given to the infant. Margie had received a saddle anesthetic and was awake during the entire procedure.

2. What kinds of fears and concerns would you expect Margie to have as she approaches her second labor-delivery experience? (List five.)

a. <u>Concern about normal development and health of her infant</u>

b. <u>Fear of long drawn out labor</u>

c. <u>Fear of lossing control</u>

d. _____

e. <u>financial concers</u>

192

3. Explain what five factors are considered when one is determining an Apgar score and how the score is determined. Complete the following chart, including an interpretation of the total score.

New name	Traditional sign	0	1	2
A apperance				
P pulse				100
G. Grimace				
A - activity				
R. Respiratory effort				

Severely depressed <u>0-3</u>

Moderately depressed <u>4-6</u>

Perfect score <u>10</u>

159

4. Margie felt well. In fact, she seemed to have more energy than usual. After preparing some frozen dinners for her husband and son to use while she was hospitalized, she decided to mop the kitchen floor and finish up a little bit of washing and ironing. She went to bed about 10:45 pm, tired but content. At 4:00 am she awoke feeling a contraction. What subtle warning of impending labor did Margie have?

<u>Sudden burst of energy</u>

159

5. What are two other indications of approaching labor that she probably experienced with her first baby but might not observe with subsequent pregnancies?

a. _lightening_

b. _engagement app. 2 weeks before._

160

6. A woman who is expecting her second child and who lives rather close to hospital facilities usually is told when contacting her physician to go to the hospital when any of the following signs of the commencement of labor have occurred (list three):

a. _Bloody show_

b. _Rapture of bag_

c. _Steady Contraction at 10-15 minutes intervals for 1 hour_

178-180

7. Margie was admitted to the hospital at 6:45 PM. Her membranes had ruptured with a gush of clear fluid in the car on the way to the hospital. Her husband, John, a teacher scheduled to be at work at 8:00 AM, had called in to school hoping to get a substitute so he could be with Margie, as planned, during most of her labor and delivery. John Jr. was staying with a kind neighbor until his grandmother could come get him. Margie was glad to receive a cordial welcome at the maternity unit and was not aware that she had arrived at that inopportune time called the "change of shift." Her contractions were coming about every 5 minutes and were lasting approximately 30 to 40 seconds. She was disappointed to learn that her cervix was dilated only about 3 cm. Using the chart on pp.80-81 as a guide, indicate the basic physical and psychological changes manifested by a typical multipara during the four stages of labor and what patient activity, nursing care, and medical supervision and intervention may be indicated.

176-177

8. Throughout her labor Margie had John's support in an LDRP. What kinds of aid can a husband or labor coach render in such a situation? (Identify three.)

a. _Giving pelvic support_

b. _Massage_

c. _mouth care, companionship & encouragement_

177, 181, 182

9. How can the nurse enhance this couple's efforts? (List three.)

a. _Giving complementary support_

b. _Teaching & reinforcing as much as possible what the_

ple had learn

c. _____

The Typical Normal Patient in Labor (see question 7 and text pp. 178-180)

Stages of labor	Physical and psychologic characteristics of the patient, contraction patterns	Suggested patient activity, including possible relaxation and breathing techniques	Recommended nursing care, common physician orders, admission procedures medications
STAGE I Cervical dilation to _10 cm_ Time range Primip _10-12 hrs_ Multip _6-8 hrs_		If membranes not ruptured	Admission procedures
Early labor _0_ to _4_ cm		If membranes ruptured	Follow-up nursing responsibilities
Midlabor _4_ to _8_ cm			Follow-up nursing responsibilities
			Other possible physician orders or nursing responsibilities
Transition _8_ to _10_ cm			Scheduled nursing responsibilities

	Scheduled nursing responsibilities	Possible anesthesia offered	
STAGE II From _Complete dilation_ To _Birth of baby_ **Time range** Primip _30 min – 2 hrs_ Multip _20 min 1½ hrs_			
STAGE III From _Birth of baby_ To _Expulsion of placenta_ **Time range** Primip _5–30 min_ Multip _5–30 min_			
STAGE IV Time Range _____			

166

10. Margie's baby was in LOA position. Indicate the area where the fetal heart rate (FHR) could be heard best by marking an X at the appropriate place on Fig. 11-1.

Fig. 11-1

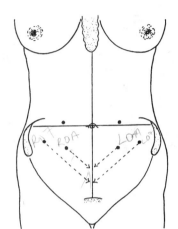

168, 170

11. What range usually is considered normal for an FHR? _____ 120-160 beats/min

When is the FHR best determined manually? _____

_____

_____

_____

172-173

12. In the light of her first labor experience, Margie was very interested in the possibility of continuous fetal monitoring. The labor room staff had just attended a conference regarding the use of the new monitoring equipment, and Margie's doctor and nurses were glad to be able to attach the internal FHR and external contraction pattern monitors on such a willing patient. Margie confided later that she found the monitors both a blessing and a nuisance. If Margie's electronic monitors had shown the following patterns, what problem if any might have been present and what intervention indicated? (See Fig. 11-2.)

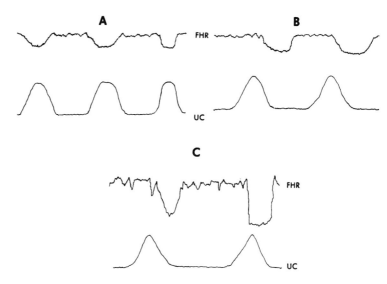

Fig. 11-2. Classic fetal heart rate and contraction patterns.

	Type of deceleration	**Problem**	**Intervention**
a.			
b.			
c.			

172-173, Fig. 11-12

176   13. Many different techniques are used to help cope with labor. Using diagrams with explanatory symbols, illustrate the following suggested breathing techniques as they are presented in the text.
          a. Deep chest or abdominal breathing (used in early and midlabor)

176   b. Accelerated-decelerated shallow panting

176   c. Pant/blow breathing (used during transition)

177   d. Describe two types of pushing that may be used during second-stage labor and explain why.

175, 177   e. Define the following terms: (1) cleansing breath, (2) focal point, (3) effleurage.

189

14. John and Margie's lively, red-haired, 8-lb baby girl was born at 11:55 AM shortly after Margie received a pudendal block and a midline episiotomy. On Fig. 11-3, indicate the line of incision for a mediolateral and a midline (or median) episiotomy.

Fig. 11-3

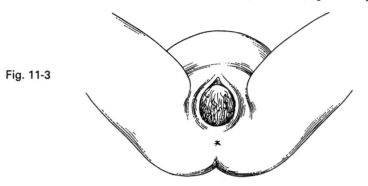

15. Following Lucinda's birth, John, Margie, and Lucinda were able to share a meaningful interval together. Later on that evening, 2-year-old John Jr. came to visit his mom and baby sister. What type of maternity care would you like to have if you were adding a child to your family?

165

16. Study Fig. 11-3, p. 165 in text. Describe how each of the measurements below may be defined, manually evaluated, and described.
   a. Duration: *from the beginning of one contraction to the end*

   b. Intensity: *the degree of peak contraction*

   c. Interval or frequency: *beginning of one contraction to the beginning of the next*

   d. Relaxation time or period: *— period between contract.*

   e. Resting tone:

164

17. External and internal uterine sensors are also helpful in detecting patterns related to fetal distress, abnormal uterine function, and placental problems, but electronic

monitoring should not be used in place of _____

_____.

196-197

18. A precipitous vertex birth: Putting things in order. Scenario: It is the last day of your student assignment on the perinatal unit. You know that all signal lights must be answered promptly. As you open the door to LDR-4 you hear the multiparous Mrs. Quick cry out, "It's coming!" And it is, the baby is crowning! (See text Fig. 11-21, p. 190) Put the following thoughts and actions in the right order, placing "Help arrives" at the bottom of the list. The first few choices and the last step have been done for you.

  1   a. Try to remain calm (appearing); think

_____ b. Use the sterile clamps and scissors carefully; otherwise there is no reason to cut the cord until much later.

_____ c. Put on sterile gloves or hold clean or sterile towel against top of infant's head with one hand.

_____ d. Suction the infant's mouth, if possible

_____ e. Feel if the cord is around the back of the baby's neck

_____ f. Try to slip the cord (if present) over the infant's head; only if it were too tight would one...

_____ g. Maintain head flexion gently and allow infant's head to deliver relatively slowly against your hand

_____ h. Tell mother to open her mouth and pant

  2   i. Activate the call light, emergency code, or intercom

_____ j. Instruct the mother firmly not to push

_____ k. Allow the infant's head to deliver between contractions while mother pants or lightly bears down

_____ l. Pinch or tear the bag of waters if it isn't already broken

_____ m. Wipe off infant's face

_____ n. Try to support the mother's perineum with your other hand

_____ o. Suction infant's nose, if possible

_____ p. Open the emergency pack in the room, if there is time

  17   q. Help arrives!

Mrs. Polly Long, a 20-year-old, is admitted at 11:30 AM in early labor with her first child. Her contractions began 2 hours before and are now 5 minutes apart lasting 30 to 45 seconds. Polly is apprehensive and appears to have little knowledge of the processes of labor and delivery. She has been under a local physician's care for 2 months. Her pregnancy appears to be physically normal. Her husband works on a construction project several miles away.

Polly was brought to the hospital by a concerned neighbor. During the admission procedures she asks that pain medication be given so that she will not lose control and be ashamed of her actions. She asks if it hurts when the bag of waters ruptures and wants to know when the doctor will "put her to sleep." The following questions relate to Polly's nursing care. Be ready to support your responses by oral discussion. Choose the one best answer.

180-182

19. To help Polly and other similar patients face their labors with more confidence:
   a. You explain everything you do in detail, including the reasons each nursing procedure is performed and what problems may develop
   b. You explain simply the labor sequence and each procedure done, emphasizing what Polly will feel and how it will help her or her baby
   c. You give her a rapid but thorough course in childbirth education
   d. You explain that everything will be all right and that she should trust her physician and not worry

179

20. Like most labor patients, Polly is encouraged to remain on her side when it is possible during labor. A lateral position is favored for all of the following reasons *EXCEPT*:
   a. Providing better fetal oxygenation
   b. Preventing maternal hypotension
   c. Promoting maternal urinary function
   d. Assisting with fetal monitoring techniques

181

21. Later the physician arrives and wants to perform a vaginal examination and possibly rupture the bag of waters. You assist the physician and help Polly undergo the examination by:
   a. Raising the head of her bed 45 degrees
   b. Checking the pH of the amniotic fluid to determine alkalinity
   c. Explaining that she will feel pressure and perhaps a gush of warm liquid
   d. Evaluating the maternal heart rate soon after the amniotic fluid appears.

181

22. The vaginal examination reveals that Polly is now dilated 5 to 6 cm and that her baby is at station O. Dr. O'Brian performs an amniotomy and attaches an internal fetal heart monitor lead to the baby's scalp. Which one of the findings below may have prompted the use of the internal monitoring technique?
   a. Contraction lasting 50 seconds
   b. Relaxation period of 2 minutes
   c. Meconium-stained fluid
   d. Complete effacement

182

23. Polly becomes alarmed when she notes an increase of reddish vaginal discharge and states that she needs the bedpan so she can move her bowels. You tell her that probably:
    a. Her bag of waters has broken
    b. Her dilation and baby's head are advancing
    c. The baby will be born within the hour
    d. She can now push effectively

182

24. The second stage of labor is characterized by:
    a. The period of transition
    b. Expulsive uterine contractions and use of abdominal musculature
    c. A relative shortening of contraction duration
    d. Increased cervical dilation

177

25. You instruct Polly in natural pushing techniques designed to avoid the fetal hypoxia sometimes associated with vigorous pushing patterns. Natural pushing includes all but which of the following?
    a. Using any position required by the woman in labor
    b. Bearing down only when the urge to push is present
    c. Bearing down against a closed glottis
    d. Pushing no longer than 5 to 6 seconds before taking another breath

189, 197

26. Polly pushed in her labor room until the small dark head of her baby was seen clearly at the vaginal opening. Then she was transferred to a delivery room. When correctly setting up the delivery room earlier, you performed all of the below EXCEPT:
    a. Placing Piper forceps on the sterile table
    b. Checking dates on sterile packages
    c. Determining the patient's Rh status and decisions regarding anesthesia and breast-feeding
    d. Consulting the doctor's equipment preferences and obtaining needed supplies

189

27. Dr. O'Brian, Polly's physician, delivered her baby Tom 20 minutes after administering saddle (spinal) anesthesia. A midline episiotomy was performed before outlet forceps were applied. Apgar scores of 7 and 8 were obtained. Polly was amazed that she did not feel the pain when the episiotomy was done or when her son was born. The routine use of episiotomies and outlet forceps is controversial. However, at times to shorten the time of expulsion and/or avoid perineal laceration they may be beneficial. All of the following related statements are true EXCEPT:
    a. First and second degree lacerations exclude the rectal sphincter
    b. A syringe, anesthetic, various needles, suture and sponges will be needed for Polly's repair
    c. Following repair an ice pack may be ordered to prevent swelling
    d. Inadequate obstetric repairs can lead to problems in the postpartal period or later in life

198   28. Some women have appointments for their infants' births. However, there must be substantial reason for artificially beginning or inducing labor, certain conditions usually must be present, and the possible problems of the procedure must be recognized. The greatest risk of oxytocin- (Pitocin) induced labor is:
    a. Uterine infection
    b. Uterine hyperstimulation
    c. Precipitous delivery
    d. Maternal hypertension

198   29. The current rate of cesarean births approximates 20% in the United States. Which has been the most frequent indication cited for the surgery?
    a. Poor progress in labor
    b. Breech presentation
    c. Previous cesarean
    d. Fetal distress

199   30. When compared to the birth of a single infant, the birth of twins is associated with a greater incidence of all the following *EXCEPT*:
    a. Malpresentation
    b. Postmaturity
    c. Placenta previa
    d. Maternal hemorrhage

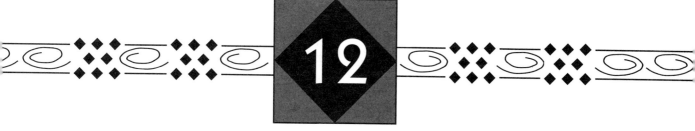

Pharmacological Pain Management

Page Reference

203

1. Define each of the following terms as it is used in obstetrics.

a. Amnesic _____

_____

b. Analgesic _____

_____

c. Hypnotic _____

_____

d. Tranquilizer _____

_____

e. Anesthetic _____

_____

f. Agonist _____

_____

g. Antagonist _____

_____

2. Fill in Table 12-1

Frequently Used Pharmacological Pain Management Options During Labor and Birth in the USA		
First Stage Labor	**Principal Advantages & Duration**	**Principal Disadvantages**
Types of Systemic Analgesia	**State duration of effective analgesia (Items a, b, c, d)**	
1. Narcotics a. meperidine (Demerol) b. fentanyl (Sublimaze)	a. b.	List 3 special concerns: (Items a, b)
2. Agonists/antagonists c. butorphonol (Stadol) d. nalbuphine (Nubain)	c. + State 1 special benefit: d. + List 2 benefits:	List 3 special concerns (Items c,d)

205
205

Frequently Used Pharmacological Pain Management Options During Labor and Birth in the USA - Cont'd		
First Stage Labor	**Principal Advantages & Duration**	**Principal Disadvantages**
Types of Systemic Analgesia		

3. Tranquilizers (potentiators)
 	
  e. promethazine (Phenergan)
 	
  f. hydroxyzine (Vistaril)
	List 3 benefits and duration: (Items e, f)	No disadvantages noted in text

Regional analgesia/ anesthesia	**Describe state of mother: (3 aspects)**	**List 6 special concerns or needs**
4. Lumbar epidural block (injection of local anesthetic, e.g., bupivacaine (Marcaine) lidocaine (Xylocaine)		
Second and Third Stages (Vaginal Birth)	**Principal Advantages**	**Principal Disadvantages**
4. Lumbar epidural block (cont'd)	List 3 benefits:	List 2 concerns : Indicate 2 rare but serious complications:

205

210-212

210-212

	Frequently Used Pharmacological Pain Management Options During Labor and Birth in the USA - Cont'd		
	Second and Third Stages (Vaginal Birth)	**Principal Advantages**	**Principal Disadvantages**
208-210	5. Subarachnoid (spinal, saddle) block (injection of local anesthetic as above)	List 3 benefits:	List 6 special concerns/needs: Indicate 1 rare but serious complication:
211-212	6. Epidural and subarachnoid with local anesthetic and *narcotics* e.g., Duramorph and/or fentanyl or sufentanil	Indicate main advantage:	List 3 side effects of method: Indicate 1 rare but serious complication:
212	7. Pudendal block with local anesthetic injected into areas just below pudendal plexus	Safety: Main use:	List 2 concerns:

204
     3. How can an institution and individual nurses help relieve pain using nonmedical means? Indicate six ways:

a. _Maintain a clean, pleasant environment_

b. _Teach & reinforce methods of relaxation_

c. _Welcome supportive companionship of those she loves._

d. _Continue to encourage her_

e. _Help the position changes and application of counter pressure_

f. _____

Although not presented in this chapter, all perinatal nurses should be knowledgeable regarding nonpharmacological methods of coping with childbirth and the basic content of such courses offered. Today, in the United States, many mothers use psychoprophylactic techniques during part of their labors and a few complete the entire process without medication.

204
     4. Special proteins called endorphins have been identified in the blood, which appear to reduce sensitivity to pain. The level of endorphins falls in the presence of all of the following body states *EXCEPT*:
a. Fatigue
b. Anxiety
c. Tension
d. Trust

204-205
     5. All the following factors influence the effect that a medication given to a laboring mother exerts on a newborn infant *EXCEPT*:
a. Amount of the drug administered
b. When, in relation to the time of birth, the drug is given
c. The presentation and position of the fetus
d. The ability of the fetus to excrete or detoxify the drug

205-206
     6. A medication that is designed to counteract respiratory depression in the newborn caused by narcotics given to a mother during labor is:
a. Phenobarbital (Luminal)
b. Naloxone hydrochloride (Narcan)
c. Methadone hydrochloride (Dolophine)
d. Epinephrine (Adrenalin)

205   7. If an analgesic or sedative is given early in labor during the latent phase, it might:
            a. Not be effective
            b. Delay or stop labor
            c. Cause teratogenic effects
            d. Cause neonatal respiratory distress

206   8. General anesthesia is infrequently employed today because:
            a. Most general anesthetics are explosive
            b. The equipment needed is not easily available
            c. The long time it takes to complete induction
            d. The danger of airway obstruction or pneumonia

206   9. Even if a woman in labor has not eaten recently, her acidic gastric secretions may be aspirated, especially during a general anesthetic. This can cause a pneumonitis called:
            a. Handel's complication
            b. Cor pulmonale
            c. Mendelson's syndrome
            d. Marfan's syndrome

206-207   10. The nurse readying a patient for emergency surgery using nitrous oxide must be sure that all the following items are removed from the patient *EXCEPT*:
            a. Wedding ring
            b. Contact lenses
            c. Dentures
            e. Chewing gum

208   11. Subarachnoid anesthesia begins to take effect immediately after administration and reaches its maximum potency in:
            a. 3 to 5 minutes
            b. 10 to 15 minutes
            c. 20 to 30 minutes
            d. 30 to 45 minutes

209   12. Patients receiving subarachnoid anesthesia are alert and unable to feel their contractions, but they usually find it difficult to:
            a. Avoid urinary incontinence
            b. Push effectively during expulsion
            c. Control nausea and vomiting
            d. Move their arms

211   13. Patients receiving epidural anesthesia should initially labor on their sides with their heads slightly raised or in modified supine positions, tilted to the left. These positions do all of the following *EXCEPT*:
            a. Help control the level of anesthesia during the first stage of labor
            b. Avoid compression of the maternal aorta
            c. Avoid compression of the maternal vena cava
            d. Assist with vaginal or rectal examination

Postpartum

Page Reference

216-218

1. Because the natural process of labor and birth can become disturbed, the postpartum patient is evaluated carefully, especially during the 1- to 4-hour period after delivery. List nine types of observations, measurements, or areas of concern that should be considered during this early interval and why they are important.

   a.

   b.

   c.

   d.

   e.

   f.

   g.

   h.

   i.

215   2. The postpartum period or puerperium usually is considered to be

a. _____ long. During this time the organs of reproduction located in the pelvis return approximately to their state before

pregnancy. This process is called b. _____.

> This morning Mrs. Vera Fast delivered her sixth child in 14 years—a noisy 9 lb, 3 oz boy, 15 minutes after her arrival at the hospital. In spite of the size of the infant, she required no episiotomy and received no laceration. No anesthesia was given. She explained that "things began to happen quite rapidly while we were on our way." Considering her history, a gravida 6, para 6 within 14 years and the large infant just born, Mrs. Fast should be considered a likely candidate for postpartum hemorrhage.

216-217   3. What elements of the postpartum evaluation are most likely to reveal the onset of this complication? (List at least 4.)

a. _____

b. _____

c. _____

d. _____

216   4. In most cases the usual location of the top of the uterus or fundus immediately after the delivery of the placenta and the day following the birth is

_____.

225   5. Indicate five factors that can influence its position in the abdomen.

a. _____

b. _____

c. _____

d. _____

e. _____

225   6. How is the condition and location of fundus usually recorded? Explain and give an example of what a nurse would expect to chart after examining Mrs. Fast's abdomen.

216-217

7. List four preliminary interventions to cause the uterine muscles to contract and prevent or stop postpartum hemorrhage.

a. _____

b. _____

c. _____

d. _____

216

8. Describe how one should massage a relaxed, soft, or boggy fundus.

Joan Sessions 34, gravida 2, para 2, was excited and relieved when she felt her first contraction yesterday. Now 14 hours later, elated 10-year-old Alice has a 2-hour-old little brother, Alexander, whom she would meet face to face this evening. As you enter Mrs. Sessions' LDRP to introduce yourself and continue her postpartum assessment and care, you hear her say on the telephone, "Now, if I could only empty my bladder, all would be well!"

Mrs. Sessions has already been catheterized twice, once during midlabor and again just before delivery. She received a lumbar epidural block during labor. Her IV containing Pitocin is infusing at 125 ml/hr. As another hour passes, there are indications again that her bladder is filling.

217

9. List 4 signs of a distended bladder.

a. _Rasiny fundus displaced to right or left_

b. _Puffy area above pubic bone_

c. _Patient complaints of feeling fullness_

d. _Dribbling_

217-218

10. List 6 ways that voiding may be encouraged.

a. _____

b. _____

c. _____

d. _____

e. _____

f. _____

219

11. You review the catheterization procedure with your instructor. In doing this procedure, you must remember to: (Circle the appropriate letter[s] below.)
    a. Check to determine if a urine specimen is needed
    b. Gain good visibility of the area by securing good lighting and parting the labial minora gently but adequately
    c. Cleanse the vestibule meticulously, using up and down scrubbing motions
    d. Lubricate the catheter and insert it approximately 6 inches into the urethra

> You secure the "cath kit." Then Mrs. Sessions announces that her legs no longer feel numb and lifts them both easily over the side of the bed. You take her blood pressure, which remains steady. This is just what the doctor ordered! You and your instructor help her to the toilet for a measured void. Soon Mrs. Sessions calls out, "It's working!" The total amount voided is 550 ml. You help her with her perineal care, instructing her what to do. No urine specimen is needed. With your aid she returns to bed. Her fundus is firm, midline below the umbilicus. You cancel the catheterization kit charge. You sigh—are you relieved because it wasn't needed or disappointed that you didn't get the learning experience?

225-226

12. Why is pericare performed (4) reasons

    a. _____

    b. _____

    c. _____

    d. _____

> Mrs. Sessions has decided to formula-feed Alex because she will be returning to work after 6 weeks. She remembers how uncomfortable her breasts were a few days after her first child was born.

222

13. What is meant by breast engorgement?

223

14. What can she do to ease this problem? (Cite 4 ways)

    a. _____

    _____

    b. _____

    _____

c. _____

_____

d. _____

_____

222

15. Do breast-feeding mothers have this problem? What can they do? (Cite 4 options)

a. _____

_____

b. _____

_____

c. _____

_____

d. _____

_____

Diane Dunlap, 22, gravida 2, para 2 has just been transferred from the Post Anesthesia Care Unit (PACU) after undergoing a repeat cesarean birth by appointment. Two years ago she had an emergency section as the result of fetal distress secondary to a prolapsed cord. The surgery was a success, but tragically Bob Jr. did not survive infancy, dying of complications of congenital heart disease. This pregnancy has been a bitter-sweet period in the lives of Diane and her husband. Currently, Diane notes many differences between the rapid, tense, frightening previous experience and her current situation. She appreciates being in a mother-baby unit and the fact that her family members are welcome to visit baby Donna and herself.

229-231

16. Indicate 10 ways that the needs or care of a cesarean-birth mother differ from those of women who have had a vaginal birth. A new postpartum patient who has had a cesarean needs:

a. _____

_____

b. _____

_____

c. _____

_____

d. _____

_____

e. _____

_____

f. _____

_____

g. _____

_____

h. _____

_____

i. _____

_____

j. _____

_____

235   17. Diane shared with her night nurse some of the ways they tried to cope with the loss of their son. When parents face the grief of an imperfect, ill, or dead child, what can be done by the perinatal staff to help ease grief and loss? (Give 3 examples.)

222   18. Early ambulation offers all the following patient benefits *EXCEPT*
   a. Decreases vaginal flow
   b. Helps prevent constipation
   c. Reduces incidence of thrombophlebitis
   d. Promotes the return of strength

217   19. During the first four hours after birth, heavy vaginal drainage has usually been defined as:
   a. Saturation of 1 tampon in $1/2$ hour
   b. Saturation of 1 peripad in 1 hour
   c. Saturation of 2 peripads in 1 hour
   d. Lochial drainage on the underpad

225   20. The first vaginal drainage after birth is normally:
   a. Lochia rubra
   b. Lochia serosa
   c. Lochia alba
   d. No special sequence

227   21. A perineal laceration involving the skin, mucous membrane, and muscles of the
                   true perineum and anal sphincter is considered what degree?
                   a. 1st degree
                   b. 2nd degree
                   c. 3rd degree
                   d. 4th degree

225-227   22. Postpartal perineal cleansing involves all of the following concepts *EXCEPT*:
                   a. Such care is essentially the same in principle whether given by nurse or patient
                   b. Any equipment used by one person should not be used by another unless
                      sterilized
                   c. Douching is an acceptable addition to postpartum hygiene
                   d. Peripads are applied/removed from front to back, following the "clean to dirty"
                      concept

227   23. Because their earlier use may cause greater bleeding, perineal heat lamps and sitz
                   baths are usually not offered after birth until how many hours have passed?
                   a. 6
                   b. 8
                   c. 10
                   d. 12

227   24. Perineal lamps must be positioned no closer to the perineum than:
                   a. 12 in
                   b. 18 in
                   c. 24 in

227   25. An antiseptic-analgesic perineal spray, if ordered, should be applied _____
                   the heat treatment.
                   a. before
                   b. after

225   26. During the early postpartal period when uterine involution is especially evident,

                   breast-feeding mothers and _____ are likely to have so called "afterpains."
                   a. Primiparas
                   b. Multiparas
                   c. Athletes
                   d. Teenagers

225   27. When a breast-feeding baby starts sucking, oxytocin from the posterior pituitary is
                   released, allowing milk to flow to the milk duct reservoirs to be ready for the
                   infant. This action is called:
                   a. Homan's sign
                   b. The sucking reflex
                   c. The let-down reflex
                   d. The rooting reflex

232   28. Many new mothers experience a transitory depression that includes tearfulness,
                   unexplained sadness, irritability, and other disturbances. These symptoms may be
                   indicative of more serious psychiatric problems especially if they last more than:
                   a. Two weeks
                   b. Four weeks
                   c. Two months
                   d. Six months

1. Encouraged by those clients and caregivers seeking a more natural, less regimented prepared participation in the process of normal labor and birth, some previously common techniques employed involving a woman's positioning, breathing, and pushing patterns have been undergoing considerable study and revision. For this type of childbirth more freedom in the selection of labor postures is being advocated. Protracted periods of directed pushing just because the cervix is completely dilated are now considered counterproductive and potentially damaging. What is being suggested? Why?

REFERENCES

Biancuzzo M: Six myths of maternal posture during labor, *MCN* 18(5):264-269, 1993

Cosner KR and de Jong E: Physiologic second-stage labor, *MCN* 18(1):38-43, 1993.

Janke J: Teaching breathing techniques in the 90's, *Internat J Childbirth Ed* 7(2):33-35, 1992

2. The growing use of epidural anesthesia in the perinatal setting as a method of pain relief during labor and delivery in the 1980s and 90s has had a significant impact on the care of many childbearing women in the United States. This "high-tech" approach to maternity provides certain desirable advantages but also involves some drawbacks. What are some of the pluses and minuses to consider when evaluating this method of pain control? What have been reactions of childbirth educators?

REFERENCES

International Childbirth Education Association, Inc.: *ICEA position paper:* epidural anesthesia for labor, Minneapolis, Minn, Nov 1987.

Simchak M: Epidurals still on the rise—is childbirth education necessary anymore? *Internat J Childbirth Ed* 6(2):37,1991.

Smith DS: Remaining strong and true in a climate of change, *Internat J Childbirth Ed* 6(2):17-18, 1991.

Taylor T: Epidural anesthesia in the maternity patient, *MCN* 18(2):86-93, 1993.

Wild L and Coyne C: The basics and beyond: epidural analgesia, *AJN* 92(4):26-36, 1992.

3. "Postpartum blues" is a common phrase and a frequent occurrence. Less common but much more serious are the possibilities of a more sustained depression or postpartum psychosis, diagnoses that the nursing staff should not forget, although they may not see the signs and symptoms during the patient's brief hospital stay. What are some cues of impending neuroses or more serious emotional problems a nurse may detect? What can be done?

REFERENCES

Affonso DD et al: Pregnancy and postpartum depressive symptoms, *J Women's Health* 2(2)157-164, 1993.

Jones LC: Postpartum emotional disorders, ICEA Review 14(4) in *Internat J Childbirth Ed* 5(4):21-28, 1990.

Kendall-Tackett KA and Kantor GK: *Postpartum depression—a comprehensive approach for nurses,* Newbury Park, Calif, 1993, Sage Publications.

Martell LK: Postpartum depression as a family problem, *MCN* 15(2):90- 93, 1990.

4. In 1992 breast-feeding was initiated by approximately 54% of mothers in the United States. Studies suggest that many women who return to the workplace would welcome more help in maintaining breast-feeding after their maternity leave ends. What suggestions do these references include?

REFERENCES

Auerbach KG: Assisting the employed breast-feeding mother, *J Nurse Midwifery* 35(1):26-34, 1990.

Dimico G: Teaching breast-feeding to working mothers, *Internat J Childbirth Ed* 6(2):20-21, 1991.

Greenberg CS and Smith K: Anticipatory guidance for the employed breast-feeding mother, *J Pediatric Health Care* 5(4):204-266, 1991.

Hills-Bonczyk SG et al: Women's experiences with combining breast-feeding and employment, *J Nurse Midwifery* 38(5):257-266, 1993.

Lee N and Edwards M: An employed mother can breast-feed when, Minneapolis, Minn, 1991, ICEA/Pennypress.

Queenan JT, editor: Breast-fed is still best-fed, *Contemp OB/GYN* 38(2):6,9, 1993.

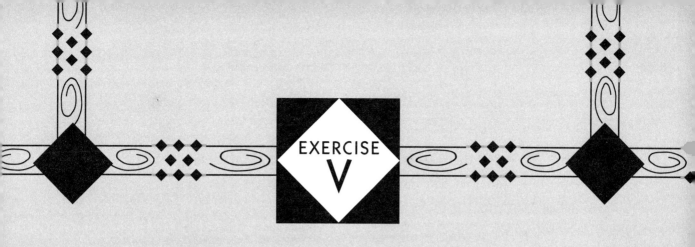

EXERCISE V

SPECIAL SITUATIONS IN CHILD-BEARING

Although pregnancy, labor, and delivery are normal physiological functions on which the human race depends for its continuity, deviations from the norm can, nevertheless, occur. A notable number of women encounter significant medical-surgical, psychosocial, or obstetrical difficulties that may greatly influence their experience of motherhood. These next two chapters discuss briefly some of the more common problems seen and what health care providers may do to help prevent, cure, or lessen the troubles they represent.

CLINICAL TIE-IN

1. Review the obstetrical histories of the patients you have cared for this week. How many would you place in the increased risk category? Why?

2. Write a nursing care plan for an obstetrical patient you contacted who had an abnormal labor and delivery or a particular health problem during her pregnancy or postpartum period.

3. What policies regarding the care of grieving mothers (those with ill, deformed, or stillborn infants) do you identify in the facility where you receive your obstetrical experience?

4. What resources for obstetrical care, preparation for child-bearing, learning child-care skills, counseling, and continued schooling are available in your community for teenage mothers and fathers?

5. During your perinatal nursing experience have you met any primigravidas 35 years of age or older? What kind of concerns did they indicate regarding their pregnancies?

Some Conditions or Characteristics That Consitute Increased Risk For a Mother and Her Unborn Child

1. Low socioeconomic, educational status (influencing especially nutrition, prenatal care supervision, and compliance)
2. Little or no prenatal care
3. Maternal age less than 18 or more than 35 years old
4. More than four pregnancies (especially if more than 35 years old)
5. Conception within 2 months of last delivery
6. Living at high altitude
7. The presence of coincidental maternal disease or significant health problems involving
   a. Cardiovascular disease
   b. Renal disease
   c. Diabetes mellitus
   d. Tuberculosis or other pulmonary disease
   e. Herpes simplex, syphilis, viral infections
   f. Hereditary anomaly or possible carrier state (e.g., sickle-cell anemia, myelomeningocele, cystic fibrosis, osteogenesis imperfecta)
   g. Use of drugs: alcohol, nicotine, and street drugs
   h. Ingestion of fetotoxic medication, exposure to radiation or toxic chemicals

i. Obesity (more than 20% greater than standard weight for height)
8. Previous obstetric complications that may recur, such as
   a. Preeclampsia-eclampsia (pregnancy-induced hypertension)
   b. Severe anemia, clotting problems, intrapartum or postpartum hemorrhage
   c. Cephalopelvic disproportion
9. Previous poor fetal outcome (repetitive fetal loss, stillbirth)
10. Deviations in the current pregnancy such as
   a. Twinning or other multiple pregnancies
   b. Premature or small-for-date fetus
   c. Postmature fetus (more than 42 weeks)
   d. Breech presentation
   e. Polyhydramnios or oligohydramnios
   f. Preterm or prolonged rupture of membranes
   g. Any of the complications noted in Section 8 above
   h. Obstetric complications (placenta previa, abruptio placentae, abnormal presentation, Rh or blood group sensitization)

Complications
of Childbearing

Page Reference

243

1. Increased risk of complications during pregnancy, birth, and the postpartum period may involve psychosocial (PS) concerns, medical (M) findings, or obstetrical (O) deviations from normal. Using the box listing high risk factors for a mother and her unborn child, place the code letters (PS), (M), or (O) in the margin next to the number or small letter groupings to indicate the types of increased risk the categories or groupings represent. (Some groupings may actually represent more than one type of increased risk.) Write your evaluations below in the box provided. Two sample partial answers have been illustrated to help you understand the placement of your answers.

(PS) 1.	6.
2.	(M) 7. g, h, i=(M)(PS)
3.	8.
4.	9.
5.	10.

2. Medical problems present before the advent of pregnancy or surfacing during gestation may pose particular problems for the infant and the mother. Examples are diabetes mellitus (considered later in Clinical Situation 2) and the following other conditions:

246
   a. Cardiac disease:
     (1) What do the designations Class III and Class IV indicate about the severity of the disease?

(2) At what three times during pregnancy does maximum cardiac stress typically occur?

(3) Five signals of cardiac overload or decompensation would be:

247

b. Urinary problems:
(1) Three indications of bladder infection are:

(2) Four indications of kidney infection are:

(3) Untreated infection or chronic or advanced renal disease may cause:

247-248

c. Tuberculosis
(1) Four general symptoms are:

(2) Four pulmonary symptoms are:

(3) Treatment of pregnant mother with active disease usually consists of:

(4) Protective medication for newborn consists of:

3. Following are completion questions highlighting seven STDs that can have a significant negative effect on the outcome of pregnancy. The impact of STDs depends on the specific infection(s) involved, the state of health of the mother and developing child, the recognition and treatment of the disease(s), and the length of the pregnancy.

248
   a. Infection in the first trimester may cause: (list 2 problems)

_____ or _____

248
   b. Infection in later pregnancy may result in: (list 3 problems)

_____   _____

_____ and/or the continued illness of the mother and/or newborn. The ability of a woman to have future children may be impaired. All of these STDs may be at times infectious but asymptomatic.

248-249
   c. Syphilis: organism: *Treponema pallidum*

     (1) The characteristic lesion or sore that forms at the portal of entry of the

spirochaete is called a _____.

     (2) The second stage of the disease may be identified by the transient presence of two types of skin lesions. Describe both.

_____

_____

_____

     (3) Three other signs or symptoms of this stage are: _____

_____

_____

     (4) Unless treated successfully the disease will progress to the third stage

characterized by: _____

_____

_____

     (5) Four signs of congenital syphilis at birth are: _____

_____

_____

_____

     (6) Modes of transmission (List 5):

_____

_____

_____

_____

_____

(7) Syphilis may be detected by two means: _____

_____ and _____ .

(8) Adequate treatment with _____ in the first
or second stages of syphilis brings optimistic prognosis.

249-250   d. Gonorrhea: organism: *Neisseria gonorrhoeae*

(1) Caused by a diplococcus, the two primary indications of the infection by sex
are:

Female	Male
_____	_____
_____	_____

(2) Continuing infection may cause: (List four possible effects for male, female,
or newborn.)

_____

_____

_____

_____

(3) Medical therapy may be complicated because:

_____

250   e. Chlamydia: organism: *Chlamydia trachomatis* (CT)

(1) Caused by a bacterium, this disease is the _____
STD in the United States today, easily surpassing gonorrhea, which shares
some of its characteristics and outcomes.

(2) It is recommended that patients with either chlamydia or gonorrhea receive

treatment for _____ .

(3) A newborn may be infected as he or she passes through the birth canal

and may demonstrate _____ .

and/or _____ .

250-251   f. Herpes genitalis: organisms: Herpes simplex virus types 1 and 2

(1) Caused primarily by Herpes simplex virus type 2, (HSV-2).

(2) The primary episode of genital blisters typically is accompanied by other
signs and symptoms: (List 3)

_____

_____

_____

(3) It is typically more _____ and _____ than
recurrent episodes.

(4) Infected persons shed the virus _____ and _____ .

    (5) An infant born vaginally of a mother suffering from primary genital herpes

         has a _____ % chance of neonatal infection. If newborn herpes infection

         occurs, the mortality rate is over _____ % and survivors may have neurological damage.

    (6) A mother with active lesions (primary or recurrent) near term, in labor, or

         with ruptured membranes usually has a _____.

251

g. Cytomegalic Inclusion Disease (CID): organism: Cytomegalovirus (CMV)

    (1) CMV causes serious illness only in_____ and

         _____.

    (2) Transmission may occur across the placenta via infected _____

         _____ during vaginal birth, or by kissing or breast-feeding the infant.

    (3) The fetus may suffer damage or _____.

    (4) There is no satisfactory _____.

251-252

h. Human Immunodeficiency Virus Disease: organism: Human immunodeficiency virus (HIV)

    (1) May progress to _____.

    (2) In the United States two behaviors which most often cause women to become HIV + are:

         _____

         _____

    (3) Transmission of HIV to the fetus or neonate may occur in three ways:

         _____

         _____

    (4) At birth, the infant of any HIV + mother will have maternal antibodies

         against HIV lasting _____.

    (5) Not all infants of HIV + mothers are infected. Those that are infected are usually asymptomatic at birth but usually develop AIDS

         by_____ .

    (6) It is highly recommended that all pregnant women at increased risk for the

         HIV virus be screened as _____

         _____.

252

i. Hepatitis B: organism: Hepatitis B virus (HBV)

    (1) All pregnant women should be tested for _____ to detect HBV.

(2) HBV may be transmitted by contact with_____ and

_____ and_____ .

(3) The primary concern is exposure of the neonate during birth to

_____ .

(4) Infants born to mothers who have hepatitis during pregnancy should be

given _____ and the hepatitis B vaccine.

252-258, 260   4. Bleeding disorders: A common threat to mother and fetus
264-266   a. A large group of obstetric complications may cause significant bleeding.
268-271   List 8 and indicate when they occur:

First half **of pregnancy** **(list 3)**	**Second half** **of pregnancy** **(list 5)**

258   b. List at least 5 categories of nursing considerations involving admission and
                          continuing care when a maternity patient is experiencing abnormal bleeding.

252-254   c. Matching: Types of abortion

_____ spontaneous (miscarriage)	1.	total
_____ induced (therapeutic)	2.	possible
	3.	certain
_____ threatened	4.	partial
_____ inevitable	5.	delayed
	6.	planned
_____ missed	7.	unplanned
_____ recurrent	8.	successive
	9.	infected
_____ complete		
_____ incomplete		
_____ septic		

256-258

d. Contrast the two hemorrhagic conditions involving the placenta considering the anatomy involved; the predisposing factors, signs, and symptoms; and type of care.

	Abruptio Placentae (Premature Separation of Placenta)	**Placenta Previa**
Anatomy involved		
Possible predisposing factors		
Signs and symptoms		

258-264

5. The disease with many names:
   Toxemia of pregnancy (old)
   Preeclampsia eclampsia
   Pregnancy-induced hypertension (PIH)

> You are assigned the care of Nancy Poor, a pale, 20-year-old, unwed, 8 months' pregnant primipara with conspicuous edema of the face and hands, admitted yesterday to the hospital. She had come to the clinic for prenatal supervision only irregularly in spite of several public health nurse contacts and admonitions by the doctors and nurses. While attending a community college and working part time, Nancy was living away from home in a small apartment with a boyfriend. She said her parents were divorced, and because she and her mother frequently quarreled, she had not been home to live for over a year. She volunteered that she and her boyfriend were intending to marry, but "couldn't just yet." Nancy states that she has gained 35 lb during her pregnancy and believes that more than 5 lb have been added in just the last 2 weeks. She cannot understand this, because she has not "felt like eating very much lately."

258, 260

a. List four aspects of Nancy's condition or background that often are associated with preeclamptic patients.

_____

_____

_____

_____

261   b. Using the chart below (based on Table 14-3 in the text), complete descriptions of the worsening of the listed characteristics from mild to severe preeclampsia.

Characteristics	Mild Preeclampsia	Severe Preeclampsia
SIGNS AND SYMPTOMS OF PREGNANCY-INDUCED HYPERTENSION		
Blood Pressure		
Proteinuria (Albuminuria)		
Edema		
Neurological Signs and Sympotms		
Other Organ Involvement		

258, 260

c. Underline the three classic signs of (PIH) or preeclampsia on the chart. Pregnancy-induced hypertension is diagnosed if:

_____

_____

258

d. The cause of this disease is _____
   List four factors that have been considered to be involved:

_____

_____

_____

_____

260

e. List four of the categories of expectant mothers who are more likely to develop (PIH).

_____

_____

_____

_____

260

f. What two events can trigger the change of diagnosis from preeclampsia to eclampsia?

_____

261-262

g. If an expectant mother with mild preeclampsia is hospitalized, identify at least eight differences her nurse should investigate incorporating within her nursing care plan that would recognize the characteristics and risks of her pregnancy.

265

h. Drug review: magnesium sulfate.
   (1) Why is magnesium sulfate ordered for severely preeclamptic patients?

   (2) What side effects may occur? What danger signals should be anticipated? (List 4)

   (3) What drug is used for an antidote to excessive effects of magnesium sulfate?

_____

6. Premature problems: PROM, PPROM, and premature labor

266-267

   a. Define and describe dangers to mother and fetus
      (1) PROM:

      (2) PPROM:

267-268

   b. Premature Labor and Birth
      (1) Indicate four reasons to try to avoid them.

(2) Identify the two main methods used to halt premature labor. What other kinds of information, skills, or support may be needed?

271

7. Puerperal infection: Its many forms
   a. Broad definition:

   b. Four factors often considered today in defining puerperal infection are:

   c. Cite five other signs of infection other than fever when infection invades the pelvis.

256-257
265, 272

8. The most common cause of maternal death is now pulmonary embolism.
   a. Cite three complications of childbearing that may be associated with emboli.

265, 272

   b. Record five classic signs of pulmonary embolism.

After 8 years of marriage and efforts to have children of their own, which resulted in three miscarriages, Ernesto and Esperanza Estrella decided to adopt. The preliminary adoption investigations had just been completed when surprised Esperanza again became pregnant. Now at 30 years of age and receiving treatment for a diabetic condition of 6 years' duration, she faces the delivery of her first child in a matter of weeks with a mixture of delight, apprehension, and wonder.

242

9. Esperanza would be considered at higher risk than most primiparas for which of the following reasons?
   a. She has wanted a child so much
   b. She has had difficulty carrying pregnancies
   c. She is an "elderly primipara"
   d. She has gestational diabetes mellitus

244

10. Dr. Murphy is pleased with Esperanza's progress, and although there had been some problems with determining optimum insulin dosage, they seemed to diminish as the pregnancy advanced. Insulin requirements during pregnancy often fluctuate. However, in early pregnancy (until about 18 weeks' gestation) the need for insulin typically:
    a. Decreases slightly
    b. Increases markedly
    c. Remains stable

242

11. Nearly 1 in 300 pregnancies is complicated by the condition diabetes mellitus. Those mothers who show signs of diabetes only when pregnant and who receive appropriate prenatal care can expect to have:
    a. No high infant mortality than healthy mothers
    b. A higher incidence of infant mortality
    c. An increased risk of complications at delivery
    d. A lower incidence of maternal complications

245

12. Optimum home control and management of the diabetic mother includes all of the following EXCEPT:
    a. Blood glucose monitoring
    b. Urine testing for glycosuria
    c. Insulin administered subcutaneously or by infusion pump
    d. Diet and exercise modifications

245

13. To follow the condition of his two patients more closely, Dr. Murphy had Esperanza visit the antepartal testing unit after 34 weeks of gestation. Which of the following procedures would not be ordered normally for her during this period?
    a. Amniotic fluid analyses
    b. Nonstress tests
    c. Ultrasound examinations
    d. Electrocardiogram

244

14. Esperanza was scheduled for a cesarean section 3 weeks before her EDD. A 7-lb, 8-oz boy was delivered in good condition and sent to the neonatal intensive care unit (NICU) for observation. Babies of mothers who are hyperglycemic late in pregnancy usually:
    a. Are immature physiologically
    b. Are small for gestational age
    c. Suffer from hyperglycemia
    d. Have high calcium blood levels

244   15. After the birth of the baby and the expulsion of the placenta, nurses should expect that maternal need for insulin for a period of time will:
     a. Decrease abruptly
     b. Increase abruptly
     c. Remain the same
     d. Decrease gradually

242   16. Today, mothers who receive optimal care who have diabetes before pregnancy experience a perinatal mortality of about:
     a. 1%
     b. 5%
     c. 10%
     d. 15%

245   17. The goal of diabetic treatment during pregnancy is to achieve and maintain normal maternal glucose levels during a 24-hour period of:
     a. 60 to 120 mg/dl
     b. 80 to 130 mg/dl
     c. 100 to 120 mg/dl
     d. 120 to 150 mg/dl

254   18. The leading cause of maternal mortality in the first trimester of pregnancy is:
     a. Abortion
     b. Placenta previa
     c. Ectopic pregnancy
     d. Amniotic fluid embolism

255   19. Classic symptoms of ectopic pregnancy characteristically include all of the following *EXCEPT*:
     a. Lower abdominal quadrant pain
     b. Shoulder pain
     c. Massive vaginal bleeding
     e. Urge to defecate

255   20. Definitive diagnosis of the presence of hydatid mole is now usually made on the basis of:
     a. Ultrasound findings
     b. Urine hormonal titers
     c. Intrauterine biopsies
     d. Uterine growth records

255   21. A major concern related to the diagnosis of hydatid mole is developing:
     a. Intrauterine infection
     b. Tubal inflammation
     c. Fetal cleft lip and palate
     d. Intrauterine malignancy

260   22. During prenatal care visits, expectant mothers should be assessed for developing signs or symptoms of edema. Which sign or symptom is considered to be least significant?
     a. Ankle swelling
     b. Facial swelling
     c. Finger swelling
     d. Sudden weight gain

120   Complications of Childbearing

262   23. All physicians agree that the best therapy for preeclampsia is:
    a. Diuretics and a low salt, low calorie diet
    b. Complete bed rest in side-lying position
    c. Antihypertensives and frequent fetal monitoring
    d. Birth of a viable infant as soon as possible

258   24. All of the following are causes of death associated with preeclampsia-eclampsia *EXCEPT*:
    a. Aspiration pneumonia
    b. Cerebral hemorrhage
    c. Antepartal infection
    d. Cardiac failure

264   25. Examples of difficult labor (dysfunctional labor or dystocia) include all of the following *EXCEPT*:
    a. Ineffective uterine contractions
    b. Umbilical cord prolapse
    c. Fetal malpresentations
    d. Cephalopelvic disproportion

268   26. Women with threatened premature births may be given any of the medications listed below *EXCEPT*:
    a. Terbutaline sulfate (Brethine)
    b. Magnesium sulfate ($MgSO_4$)
    c. Oxytocin (Pitocin)
    d. Ritodrine (Yutopar)

268   27. If premature labor is inevitable, little analgesic medication is given (although a type of spinal anesthesia may be administered at delivery) because it can:
    a. Slow the labor
    b. Depress fetal respirations
    c. Make the mother less alert
    d. Cause fetal convulsions

271   28. In cases of puerperal infection involving the pelvis, the patient is most often asked to maintain a:
    a. Side-lying position
    b. Trendelenburg's position
    c. Sim's position
    d. Fowler's position

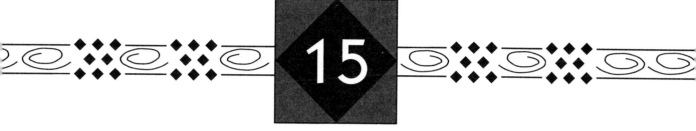

Special Needs
and Age-Related
Considerations

Page Reference

278

1. List eight factors that have been cited as causes of the increase in unwed teen pregnancy in the United States today.

278

2. Normal adolescent progress toward adulthood is characterized by advancing physical, emotional, and cognitive maturation to achieve which three psychological developmental tasks?

278-279

3. Identify three female characteristics of each of the three age divisions of adolescence indicated below:
    a. Early adolescence (12 to 15 years)

    b. Middle adolescence (15 to 17 years)

    c. Late adolescence (17 to 20 years)

279-280

4. Complete the following statements related to teenage pregnancy outcomes. In general, the younger the adolescent at the time of pregnancy and childbirth, the more

    serious the (a) _____ , _____

    risks; and the more profound the (b) _____ consequences. Because of poor quality nutrition and insufficient calories teenagers are

    at increased risk for having a (c) _____ and/or

    (d) _____ baby. The key to preventing physical complications is (e) _____ _____

    _____ begun in the (f) _____

    trimester. Single-parent families often live in (g) _____ and even those who marry are at risk for economic problems. Pregnancy and

    parenting are likely to disrupt, delay, or end the (h) _____ of young adolescent mothers (and fathers).

279

5. The economic cost of adolescent pregnancy to the nation as a whole as society attempts to help meet the needs of this special group is tremendous. Name at least four governmental programs that assist parents and children.

280　　　　6. Two national health objectives for the year 2000 involving adolescent sexual behavior are:

281　　　　7. Teenage parents do have strengths that nurses can foster. They report pleasure in the mothering role and astonishment at their baby's growth and development. How can the nurse encourage this natural interest? (Indicate 5 ways.)

281　　　　8. Enumerate 5 factors that are responsible for increasing the number of women who are delaying childbearing until their mid- thirties.

281-282　　9. Pregnancy and childbirth after 35 involve an increase in certain physical health and psychosocial risks. Identify 5 potential health problems that need special consideration.

282   10. Identify 5 psychosocial risks to an older expectant couple. Recognize that conditions may be quite different depending on whether the pregnancy was planned.

277   11. Age-related pregnancy risks have been particularly identified affecting females and their babies in the following groups:
    a. Women before 18 and over 30
    b. Women before 15 and over 30
    c. Women before 17 and over 35
    d. Women before 19 and over 35

277   12. In the United States the proportion of pregnancies occurring in the 15-to-20-year-old grouping has increased to:
    a. 1 in 8
    b. 1 in 10
    c. 1 in 15
    d. 1 in 25

277   13. Young women under 20 years of age bear approximately what percentage of out-of-wedlock births in the United States?
    a. 10%
    b. 20%
    c. 40%
    d. 46%

279-280   14. Seeking to establish a trusting teaching relationship with a pregnant adolescent, the nurse would do well to recognize all of the following EXCEPT:
    a. The need to understand the adolescent maturational process
    b. The need to listen attentively, maintaining a nonjudgmental approach
    c. The need to make decisions for her to serve her best interest and facilitate her care
    d. The need to explain procedures and her expected plan of care in a way geared to her understanding

280   15. To help change the pregnancy health habits of a pregnant teenager, it has been suggested that caregivers emphasize:
    a. The benefits gained by the adolescent
    b. The benefits gained by her developing child
    c. The benefits gained by her future family
    d. The benefits gained by society as a whole

280   16. Although prenatal care for all ages has many similarities, adolescent care stresses the identification and treatment of risks most frequent in that group, which would include all the following *EXCEPT*:
- a. Assessment of dietary habits and hemoglobin and hematocrit levels
- b. Evaluation for hypertension, edema, proteinuria
- c. Monitoring of weight gain, fundal height, sonogram results
- d. Minimizing the dangers of drug abuse and STDs

280   17. The pregnant teenager's support system is not always intact or acceptable, but ideally it would include:
- a. The involved father of her child
- b. Her parents and/or other family members
- c. Supportive adults and teen parent groups
- d. All of the above

281   18. Although the majority of first births are to women in their twenties, the number of first births to women over 30 increased in the 1980s by:
- a. 50%
- b. 80%
- c. 100%
- d. 120%

282   19. In order to be more sensitive to the concerns and needs of older couples, it is important that the nurse not:
- a. Know whether the pregnancy was planned
- b. Be aware if there were difficulties conceiving
- c. Note if there were previous spontaneous abortions
- d. Assure them that "Everything will be alright"

1. Women have cesarean deliveries because of some complications that may or may not be encountered in another pregnancy. Some women feel unfulfilled or cheated because they have not experienced a normal vaginal birth, especially if they had been "training for the event." If the mother so wishes and certain criteria are met, an increasing number of physicians are inclined to attempt a trial labor. Childbirth educators have special vaginal birth after cesarean (VBAC) classes for hopeful couples. What criteria must be met before a VBAC is attempted? What problems do cesarean births often present that can be prevented by a vaginal birth? What should labor-delivery nurses know when caring for a mother anticipating a VBAC?

REFERENCES

Afriat C: Vaginal birth after cesarean section: a review of the literature, *J Perinatal-Neonatal Nurs* 3(3):1-13, 1990.

Crawford K: Childbirth education for VBAC, *Internat J Childbirth Ed* 7(3):20, 1992.

International Childbirth Education Association, Inc.: *ICEA position statement*: cesarean section and VBAC, Minneapolis, Minn, May 1989

Reichert JA, Baron M, and Fawcett J: Changes in attitudes toward cesarean birth, *JOGNN* 22(2):159-167, 1993

2. Today, pregnant teenagers make up a special population within our society. Many are not ready for the problems of adulthood let alone those of premature parenthood. Yet most of these young mothers choose to keep their babies (often without any assistance from the infants fathers, but, in some cases, considerable help from their grandmothers). Various programs have been constructed to try to meet their numerous needs. Below are listed articles that describe certain aspects of the efforts of health care providers and educators to reach out to this vulnerable group. Which aspects of the programs described do you consider especially helpful? What suggestions would you particularly endorse or omit? How are these classes funded? How many do they serve? What kind of follow-up contacts, if any, were attempted? How are their successes or failures measured?

REFERENCES

Attendorf J and Klepacki L: Do you believe in safe sex? Do you believe in magic? *Internat J Childbirth Ed* 7(1):15-16, 1992.

Barr L and Monserrat C: *Working with pregnant and parenting teens (resource guide teacher Ed: teenage pregnancy: a new beginning),* Albuquerque, NM, 1992 New Futures.

Fleming BW et al: Assessing and promoting positive parenting in adolescent mothers, *MCN* 18(1):32-37, 1993.

Hotelling BA: What can these babies possibly learn about having babies? *Internat J Childbirth Ed* 7(4):10-11, 1992. (Suggestions for organizing the content and presentation of classes.)

Leo J: On society: learning to say no, US News & World Report, June 20, 1994, p 24.

May KM: Social networks and help-seeking experiences of pregnant teens, *JOGNN* 21(6):497-502, 1992.

Perrin KM: The 4Ms of teen pregnancy: managing, mending, mentoring, and modeling, *Internat J Childbirth Ed* 7(4):29, 1992.

Roller CG: Drawing out young mothers, *MCN* 17(5):254-255, 1992.

Stam J and Paperny DM: Computer games to enhance adolescent sex education, MCN 15(4):250-253, 1990.

Wood D: TAPP: a school-based pregnancy program that shines, Internat *J Childbirth Ed* 7(4):19-20, 1992.

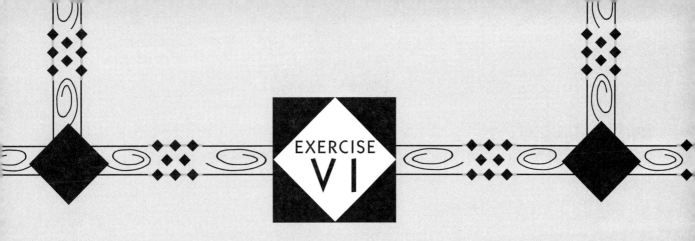

THE NEWBORN

The human newborn is unique. The young of no other species needs so much consistent care for such an extended period of time. But no other newborn has such potential or capacity to achieve. Neonatal nurses, like the parents, often may speculate what the future holds for such small, helpless appealing creatures.

Although most infants are born without any serious defect, it is estimated that approximately 1 in 14 infants has at least one kind of physical problem at birth that may manifest itself immediately or in the month and years following. This is a fairly high ratio. The problems include genetic defects, intrauterine environmental difficulties, and negative incidents associated with labor and delivery.

Newborns represent the next generation. They are indeed precious. They also can be puzzling and frightening to new parents.

CLINICAL TIE-IN

1. Keep a record of the questions that you hear asked by new mothers and fathers about their offspring. How did you or another nurse respond?

2. Watch an infant's physical examination. What observations does the health care provider make to assess gestational age; check for dislocated hip; jaundice; nervous system integrity and respiratory and cardiac function?

3. Observe how mothers relate to their infants. Do you notice signs of relaxation, warmth, competence, detachment, rigidity, tenseness, or insecurity. How do they manifest themselves?

4. How long do healthy newborns stay in the perinatal facility where you have clinical experience before going home? What implications does this information have for our community health system?

5. How many neonatal problems that you have observed could be listed as
   (1) genetic,
   (2) associated with prenatal environment, or
   (3) connected with the events of labor and delivery?

6. How many neonatal problems observed were associated with preterm birth?

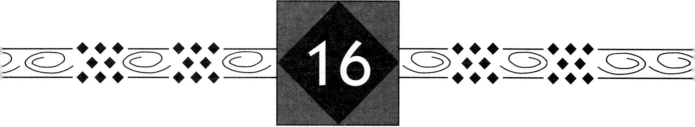

Newborn
Assessment

Page Reference

1. Add the missing information to the following vital statistics of the average newborn.

291   a. Weight (male) _____ lb _____ oz; ___3.4___ kg

291   b. Weight (female) _____ lb _____ oz; ___3.18___ kg

291   c. Length (male) ___20___ inches; _____ cm

291   d. Length (female) ___19½___ inches; _____ cm (2.54cm = 1 inch)

293   e. Head circumference (occipital-frontal OFC) _____ to _____ inches, ___33___ to ___35.5___ cm usually exceeding the diameter of the chest by 1-2 cm once molding has resolved.

290   f. Apical pulse at rest _____ to _____ /min (range)

290   g. Respirations ___30___ to ___60___ /min (range regardless of activity)

290   h. Blood pressure at birth ___80-60___ - _____ / ___45___ - ___40___

290   i. The normal range of a newborn's axillary temperature is ___97.9___ ° C or _____ ° F

2. Identify the following noteworthy newborn manifestations:

299   a. Meconium _____

_____

292   b. Vernix caseosa _____

_____

292   c. Milia ___clogged___ ___oil gland___ _____

_____

129

291

    d. Acrocyanosis _____

_____

292

    e. Lanugo _____

_____

292

    f. Stork-bites <u>Red marks seen especially at nape</u>
<u>of neck .</u>

292

    g. Mongolian or Asiatic spots _____

_____

3. Describe or explain these common abilities or behaviors of the newborn:

304

    a. Visual ability _____

_____

_____

_____

304

    b. Hearing ability _____

_____

_____

_____

304

    c. Sense of smell _____

_____

_____

304

    d. Sense of taste _____

_____

_____

304

    e. Sense of touch _____

_____

_____

301-303

    f. List 10 inborn or primitive reflexes

_____

_____

_____

_____

_____

_____

_____

_____

_____

_____

> Chris is the day-old first born of Mark and Martha Matthews. Both parents have many questions about Chris and his care.

293

4. They wonder about the rather large, spongy swelling toward the back of Chris's head, which the doctor called caput. In response to their queries you correctly state that:
   a. Caput is the result of prolonged pressure on the presenting part (head) during labor
   b. It is a collection of fluid under the periosteum of the scalp
   c. The doctor probably will aspirate the fluid from the swelling, using a sterile technique
   d. If the swelling crosses a cranial suture line, a skull fracture may be indicated

292

5. Martha is horrified to find that Chris has five or six red blotches and hivelike spots on his chest and back. With a shaky voice she calls her nurse to her bedside to see if her baby has an infection. The knowledgeable nurse looks carefully at the areas and then explains that:
   a. Until the doctor is sure what may be causing the problem, Chris should be placed in isolation
   b. She will especially note the problem but that many healthy, vigorous babies get similar rashes, which go away in time without treatment or associated problems
   c. The baby has blood poisoning
   d. Such rashes most often are seen on the extremities

291

6. Mark is concerned that Chris's feet are definitely flat. The same nurse comments that:
   a. An orthopedic specialist will be contacted if they so desire
   b. Faithful daily passive exercise to the infant's feet will cure the problem
   c. All babies are born with a fatty pad that shapes their feet in this way
   d. Chris will need to wear special supportive baby shoes

296

7. Snuggled in Martha's arms, Chris yawns widely, revealing some white, curdy material on his tongue. Overanxious, Martha thinks about a fungus problem that she had heard some babies develop. She calls you to her side. To reassure her and help clarify the problem, you would *first:*
   a. Tell her that thrush is quite easy to treat
   b. Offer some water to the baby
   c. Ask her if she has had any problem with perineal itching or a creamy-looking vaginal discharge
   d. Tell her that the same fungus may cause a diaper rash

297   8. Chris's small breast area is swollen and appears tender. This condition:
    a. Is seen only rarely in boys
    b. Indicates possible future sexual orientation problems
    c. Is called cutis marmorata
    d. Is the result of stimulation by maternal hormones

295   9. When Martha saw Chris the day after delivery, his eyelids were somewhat puffy and a small amount of drainage from his eyes was seen. All responses are correct *EXCEPT:*
    a. The eye irritation was probably the result of infection
    b. Babies occasionally experience this reaction
    c. This reaction was a response to the medication used to prevent infection
    d. The use of the medication is a legal requirement in most states

292   10. Small blue-red dots that, if present, are usually seen on the face and do not blanch on pressure are called:
    a. Stork bites
    b. Erythema toxicum
    c. Petechiae
    d. Mongolian spots

291   11. A mild yellowish cast to the skin of the newborn, which first appears about the third day after birth, usually is considered to be:
    a. A sign of gastrointestinal problems
    b. A sign of blood incompatibilities
    c. A sign of the destruction of excess red blood cells
    d. A result of a fall in serum bilirubin

290   12. A sucking-in of an infant's chest wall in the rib or sternal areas during inspiration is abnormal. These respiratory responses to poor ventilation are called:
    a. Retractions
    b. Reductions
    c. Residuals
    d. Reversals

293   13. The relatively large diamond-shaped fontanel felt on the anterior part of the baby's head normally closes by:
    a. 3-6 months
    b. 4-8 months
    c. 9-18 months
    d. 12-20 months

293   14. A bulging fontanel may indicate:
    a. Presence of severe dehydration
    b. Cardiovascular abnormalities
    c. Urinary congenital malformations
    d. Increased intracranial pressure

307   15. Which of the newborn behavior states described by T. Barry Brazelton affords an especially rewarding opportunity for parent-infant interaction?
    a. Drowsy
    b. Alert
    c. Active
    d. Crying

Care of the
Normal Newborn

Page Reference

1. Every infant has certain primary needs that must be met. These needs are supplied in various ways, depending chiefly on environmental factors and the philosophies of his caretakers. State briefly how the 10 basic needs listed below are usually supplied to an infant in our society in the follow-up evaluation period after the immediate care provided at birth.

310   a. Maintaining effective respiration (2 considerations)

(1) Suctioning excessive secretions

(2) Proper positioning the newborn on side.
   - prevent aspiration & regurgitation

311   b. Thermoregulation (5 considerations)

(1) Frequent monitoring of infants temperature

(2) Wrap infant in double warm blanket

(3) Use of radiant warmer if hypo thermia develops

(4) Prevent excessive heat loss.

311-312   c. Assessment (Besides the admission bath, physical examination, and gestational evaluation, list 3 more possible laboratory tests discussed that may be relevant)

(1) Hematocrit level.

(2) Blood glucose level for hypoglycemia or for obvious signs - jitteriness, lethargy - or temperature instability

(3) Signs of abstinence syndrome - withdrawal.

312   d. Identification and security (List 3 concurrent methods)

(1) No unattended infants

(2) Staff picture identification

(3) Referral to parent, baby wrist and ankle identification bracelets

133

312-313   e. Safe handling and positioning (5 considerations)

1. Support of head & neck needed
2. Always lift baby at 2 contact points if one fail the other is available
3. Never lift by the arms
4. Should be propped ō a rolled blanket along his back
5. Prone position no longer recommended

312-313   f. Prevention of hemorrhage (4 considerations)

1. IM vitamin K. 0.5 mg
2. Monitor cord
3. Monitor circumcision site
4. Prevent Intracranial bleeding, do not place in head-down positions for prolonged periods

314-317   g. Prevention of infection (8 considerations)

1. Meticulous staff hygiene before starting care
2. Hand washing before & after contact
3. Prophlactic eye medication
4. Monitor infant for breaks in skin
5. Antiseptic cord care and observation
6. Complete immunization

h. Nourishment (see 2 below)

324-325   i. Parent-infant interaction (List 3 ways that successful interaction may take place. Also review Chapter 16, p. 307.)

1. Need to recognize clues from infant for readiness to react
2. Clue for overstimulation
3. Realize the importance of interaction in establishing good bonding.

j. Parent education (List 4 sources of parenting information. Can you think of others not mentioned in the text?)

1. High school, college, or adult education sponsored family education class
2. Conversation with successful parents
3. Prenatal - postnatal education programs.
4. Well - child visits.

317-318

2. Susan Webb, a 26 year-old primipara has planned to breast-feed her first born, Jeffrey Webb, Jr. She made her decision when she and her husband attended a prenatal class where the advantages of breast-feeding were discussed. What are some of the benefits to her son (list 7) and herself (list 5) that she may have heard taught.

a. Helping the Mother	b. Helping the Infant
(1) Help the uterine to contract	1) Curd easier to digest than cows milk
(2) Lower risk of breast cancer	2) less likely to cause allergy
3. Provide mother & infant attachment	3) Iron content lower but better absorb
4 Delays ovulation & menstruation but no guarantee against pregnancy	4) May received immunity facts from mother
(5) Release hormone prolactin and produces a relaxing effect.	4, Lower in cholestrol
	5, Milk always fresh
	6 Babys have less respiratory tract infection

3. If it's false, make it right.
   Sometimes it's hard to remember what has been said in classes. Below are some statements related to breast-feeding that Susan remembered being discussed. If they are true, circle the T; if false, circle the F. If you mark a statement false, you must alter the statement to make it form a relevant correct sentence. Do not correct the sentence by simply making it negative.

319   T F   a. A breast-feeding mother needs an additional 500 calories per day in her diet to produce about 25 ounces of milk when lactation is fully established in the first 6 months after her infant's birth.

319   T F   b. While some nursing infants are affected by changes in their mothers' diets, no one food bothers every infant.

321   T F   c. The greatest aid to milk production is frequent stimulation and emptying of the breasts, and newborns seem to do best when allowed to nurse on demand, without limitations regarding frequency or length of feeding.

320   T F   d. To help the infant to breast-feed effectively and keep the nipple in good condition, the baby must nurse with the areola in the mouth and not just the nipple.

321   T F   e. The breasts and nipples of nursing mothers should be carefully washed with
no   mild soap, rinsed with clear water, and air dried three times (one) a day to prevent infection.

318   T F   f. Most, if not all, drugs taken by the nursing mother pass through the milk to the baby.

4. Artificial Feeding

322   a. The American Academy of Pediatrics recommends that nonbreast-fed infants

receive _iron fortified_ formula during the first year of life.

322   b. There are many infant formulas available to the shopper in the supermarkets. Some are powdered, others are concentrated liquids, and some are ready to

use. It is very important to read labels because _Improper_ _preparation can cause an infant_ _to be severely ill_

323   c. Most bottle feedings today are offered at _room_ temperature. Select appropriate nipple and be sure it is placed on top of the tongue.

323   d. Babies seem to drink best when held closely at a _45°_ .

323   e. The neck of the bottle should always be _full of milk_ .

323   f. Both breast- and bottle-fed babies must be burped because air in an infant's

stomach may (1) _pain_

(2) _decrease appetite_   (3) _promote regurgitation_

323   g. Explain how to prepare infant formula using the tap water method and the first 9 steps noted in box on p. 323.

× milk producing
gland ~ acini

324   5. Susan and her 4-day-old son Jeff seem to be doing well. The visiting postpartum nurse from the hospital is pleased with their care arrangements and health status. As usual Susan has a number of questions; one that is especially puzzling to her involves Jeff's diet. She asks, How do I know if he's getting enough milk? Discuss four main ways a newborn's intake may be evaluated.

a. *Observe behaviour*

b. *Watch for signs of dehydration*

c. *Measure intake*

d. *Measure weight gain*

310   6. Newborns may suffer from hypothermia not because they produce heat poorly, but because they are vulnerable to heat loss. All of the characteristics listed below contribute to this situation *EXCEPT*:
   a. Large body surface in relation to body weight
   b. Little subcutaneous fat for insulation
   c. Poorly developed thermoregulatory response
   d. Great reliance on the process of shivering

310   7. The newborn is aided in efforts to increase or maintain body temperature by a special tissue that helps produce heat called:
   a. Brown fat   c. Lipid layers
   b. Yellow sebum   d. Erythema

311   8. In addition to respiratory distress, the consequences of hypothermia may include hypoglycemia. Characteristic signs of hypoglycemia are all those listed below *EXCEPT*:
   a. Lethargy   c. Jitteriness
   b. Emesis   d. Temperature instability

311   9. The normal newborn hematocrit range per heel stick sample is:
   a. 30%-40%   c. 45%-50%
   b. 35%-40%   d. 45%-65%

317   10. With frequent applications of 70% isopropyl alcohol the umbilical cord is usually dry and shriveled after:
   a. 24 hours   c. 48 hours
   b. 36 hours   d. 72 hours

310   11. Before a bulb syringe is placed in the mouth of an infant to remove oral secretions, it must be:
- a. Expanded
- b. Sterilized
- c. Compressed
- d. Released

311   12. The best site for a neonate heel stick is the:
- a. Tip of the big toe
- b. Medial aspect of heel
- c. Lateral aspect of heel
- d. The back of the heel

313   13. The football hold should not be used to carry an infant because:
- a. The head is somewhat unprotected
- b. The spine is improperly supported
- c. The baby may wriggle and fall
- d. The baby's body is compressed

314   14. For 2 to 5 days following birth, the infant is at increased risk of hemorrhage because of depletion of stores of:
- a. Iron
- b. Vitamin K
- c. Vitamin E
- d. Folate

317   15. The American Academy of Pediatrics has stated that eye prophylaxis may be delayed to facilitate the initial parent-child attachment up to:
- a. 1 hour
- b. 2 hours
- c. 3 hours
- d. 4 hours

320   16. Small premature infants who may not be able to suck effectively may best benefit from breast milk given by:
- a. Cup
- b. Syringe
- c. Dropper
- d. Gavage

321   17. The first secretion from the maternal breast, particularly note for its protective antibodies and laxative effect, is termed:
- a. Witches milk
- b. Vernix caseosa
- c. Sebum
- d. Colostrum

323   18. Prefeeding or in process episodes of coughing, cyanosis, or excessive mucus are especially associated with anomalies of the:
- a. Digestive or respiratory tracts
- b. Central nervous system
- c. Musculoskeletal systems
- d. Endocrine glands

316   19. Pediatric urologists do not recommend attempting to retract the foreskin of the infant until about the age of
- a. 1 month
- b. 2 months
- c. 5 months
- d. 1 year

329   20. An infant who has been recently circumcised needs to be carefully checked for:
- a. Blood spots larger than a quarter
- b. Signs of infection or swelling
- c. Inability to urinate
- d. All of the above

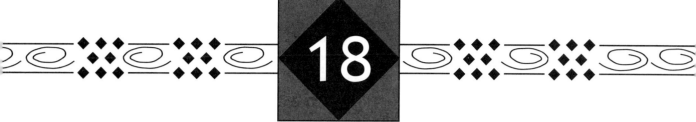

The Newborn
with Special Needs

Page Reference

334

1. Define the following terms as they apply to the newborn.

   a. Premature (preterm) _____

   _____

   b. Term _____

   _____

   c. Postterm (postmature) _____

   _____

   d. Small for gestational age (SGA) _____

   _____

   e. Low-birth-weight infants _____

   _____

   f. Very low-birth-weight (VLBW) infants *less than 1520 gm*

   _____

336

2. List four situations often associated with low-birth-weight babies.

   a. *Low socioeconomic*

   b. *Teenage pregnancy*

   c. *Multiple birth*

   d. *Excessive smoking*

   Lack of prenatal care

337

3. Contrast the appearance and other characteristics of the premature infant and the full-term infant in at least four different ways.

Characteristic	Normal newborn	Premature

342

4. List six signs of possible increasing intracranial pressure in the infant no matter what the cause (e.g., intracranial hemorrhage, tumor, abscess).

a. Vomiting

b. irritability

c. bulging of the fontanels

d. separation of cranial sutures

e. asymmetrical increase in head size

f. thinning of the skull bone.

5. Shunting is one attempt to prevent or treat hydrocephalus.

342-343

a. What types of shunts currently are being used to try to avoid or limit the development of hydrocephalus in infants? Ventriculoperitoneal shu , Lumbar-peritoneal, ventriculo atrial

343

b. Cite two problems that are associated with shunting and for which the patient must be observed.

(1) An occluded shunt no matter what the cause.

(2) an infected shunt

Approximately 2% of our population is considered to be mentally retarded. One common type of mental retardation is that associated with Down syndrome. Sally Smith is an 8-year-old child with this diagnosis. She has attended special education classes to help her meet some of her basic needs. She is able to use the toilet, bathe, dress, and feed herself, and participate in many household activities. Her parents are pleased with her progress and hope that as she gets older she will be able to work in some type of sheltered workshop. Sally is a lovable if sometime mischievous child.

349

6. List the signs of Down syndrome that you would look for when evaluating a new-born for this disorder? (Name five.)

a. _epicathic folds - which makes the eyes slant up_

b. _Short hands and fingers bent in -- Clinodactyly_

c. _Simian crease - horizontal crease across the palm_

d. _large space between the great & big toes_

e. _small white dots on iris_

349

7. Which type of Down syndrome is considered hereditary? _Translocation_

349

8. How common is Down syndrome? Are some mothers more at risk than others?

1 in 650 births . -- woman over 40 years old - near the end of their reproductivity

339-340

9. Name at least three other conditions that may be associated with mental retardation.

a. _Galactosemia_

b. _Phenylketonuria_

c. _Congenital hypothyroidism_

355

10. Erythroblastosis fetalis is a serious newborn disorder caused by a blood component incompatibility between the mother and the fetus. Fortunately, it is not common currently because a method of preventing problems associated with Rh incompatibility has been quite successful.

a. What sequence of events must take place before complications associated with the Rh factor occur?

356

b. How can the problem usually be prevented?

356

c. List four clinical manifestations of erythroblastosis.

(1) _Early jaundice_

(2) _Lethargy_

(3) _Poor sucking_

(4) _Twitching_

5, Spasticity

356   d. What treatments might be considered for the newborn who shows evidence of erythroblastosis?

Fluorecent trans fusini
exchange trans fusins

356   e. What treatment may be available to the affected fetus at certain research centers?

Intra uterine transfusion

11. Match the following abnormal newborn conditions.

358	_____ Syndactyly	a. Webbed digits
358	_____ Talipes equinovarus	b. Urethral deviation c. Extra digits
358	_____ Polydactylism	d. Rectal deviation e. Foot deformity
353	_____ Omphalocele	f. Abdominal wall defect
356	_____ Hypospadias	
353	_____ Imperforate anus	

> When young Marian Stewart became pregnant, she dreamed of having a big, energetic, "successful" son who would bring her honor and security. When Dougie finally arrived less than perfect physically, Marian had a hard time relating to the reality of the situation. Tom, her husband, was the one who seemed to hear what the physicians were saying and gently tried to help her begin to deal with the problems that were facing them as parents of a baby with a lumbar myelomeningocele.

345   12. Describe the anatomical defect "myelomeningocele" located in the lumbar area.

a protrude through the spinal opening and nerve tissue are also found in herniated sac.

345   13. List four problems that might be associated with this central nervous system abnormality and that could affect Dougie's abilities now or in the future.

a. Fecal & urinary incontenince

b. Lower extremities paralysis or weakness

c. Lower extremity loss of sensation

d. Developing hydrocephalus

345   14. The neurosurgeon called for consultation wanted to close the defect as soon as possible. Why did he elect to operate on Dougie so early in the newborn period?

To reduce the possibilety of infection

> Dougie recovered from his back surgery rapidly. His mother came in every day to see him, observe the nurses, and participate in his bath and feedings. By the time Dougie was discharged 8 days later, she was able to complete every aspect of his care. Her competence surprised both her husband and herself, and she took deserved pride in her accomplishments. The nurses complimented her and made her feel as if she could function at home with a certain amount of skill. She was glad to hear, however, that a nurse from the hospital would be able to visit her at home to answer questions and help Marian and Tom for forthcoming orthopedic procedures.

345   15. What two orthopedic defects often are associated with myelomeningocele patients?

a. Club foot

b. Dislocated hip

> Mrs. Harriet Hand was disappointed but not surprised that her baby, Holly, had a cleft lip. She had been told that there had been one child with cleft lip in each generation of her family for many years, and she herself had had a repair. She accepted the news rather philosophically.

349   16. At what age should Holly's cleft lip be repaired and why at that time?

Usually between 6-10 weeks

350   17. After the surgery you are assigned Holly's care. List two safety precautions that need to be observed during the immediate postoperative period.

a. Reduce sucking movement

b. Elbow restraint to prevent from touching

351   18. Discuss the nursing care that would be required to prevent scarring of the suture line.

337   19. Overfeeding of premature newborns must be prevented primarily because of the increased danger of:
            a. Colic
            b. Vomiting
            c. Diarrhea
            d. Fatigue

340   20. An infant with phenylketonuria must not be given foods, (e.g., cow's milk), that contain an amino acid that he or she cannot metabolize properly. This amino acid is called:
            a. Trypsin
            b. Lysine
            c. Phenylalanine
            d. Cystine

352   21. Mothers pregnant with infants who have tracheoesophageal fistula (TEF) often are found, before their deliveries, to have:
            a. High temperatures
            b. Polyhydramnios
            c. Excessive nausea
            d. Significant anemia

353   22. Which of the following *is not* a characteristic sign of the most common type of TEF?
            a. Coughing
            b. Excessive salivation
            c. Apnea
            d. Forceful vomiting

353   23. If possible, the infant with TEF is scheduled for surgery within 24 hours of birth. During the brief period before surgery, which of the following *is not appropriate* for the child?
            a. Kept in a high Fowler's position
            b. Suctioned gently by a sump tube in the esophagus
            c. Fed clear liquids by gavage
            d. Evaluated for other congenial anomalies

356   24. Newborns who have an elevated bilirubin level in their blood often are placed under fluorescent lamps. Which one of the following statements *is not included* in their care?
        a. Eyes covered when lamps on
        b. Frequent turning to expose skin surfaces
        c. Incubator care to preserve body warmth
        d. Fluid restriction enforced

357   25. The most frequently fractured bone during the birth process is:
        a. Radius
        b. Femur
        c. Clavicle
        d. Humerus

357   26. Lucy Lansing, a newborn, was found to have a congenital dislocated right hip. A true statement concerning this condition is:
        a. Prognosis with early treatment is poor
        b. Surgery is the most common method of treatment
        c. Adduction of her legs is concerned
        d. Lifting her legs for diapering is avoided

Intensive Care of the Newborn

Page Reference

362   1.   What is the main objective of the Neonatal Intensive Care Unit?

    To provide the earliest and highest degree
    of medical and nursing care of infant at risk
    so that each infant attains the possible outcome

362   2.   List the members of the neonatal transport team.

    (1) _Pediatrician_
    (2) _Neonatal nurse clinician or practitioner_
    (3) _Respiratory therapist_
    (4) _N I C U nurse_

362   3.   High-risk newborns often result from increased-risk pregnancies. List six examples
    of increased-risk pregnancies.

    a. _No prenatal care_
    b. _Poor nutrition_
    c. _Drug addiction_
    d. _P I H._
    e. _prolonged infertility_
    f. _alcholisim_

    4.   What is meant by a baby's neutral thermal range? _allows normal_
    body temperature to be maintained with the
    least expenditure of energy.

365   5. Unquestioning reliance on mechanical aids to assess an infant's well being should be discouraged, because any equipment can falter. The most important monitor of the infant is _the knowledgeable alert nurse_ .

366   6. Compared with the normal newborn, does the low-birth-weight infant need *more* or *less* calories and fluid per kilogram per day? _more_

366   7. The small vigorous infant may attempt nipple feedings if:

Intact gag and suck reflex.

370   8. List five symptoms often associated with the onset of neonatal sepsis.

a. _respiratory distress - c grunting & tachypnea_

b. _poor feeding_

c. _vommiting_

d. _lethargy_

e. _jaundice_

372   9. Unless the disease is severe and of long duration, infants of diabetic mothers are characteristically (list two features):

a. _L.G.A , hypoglycemia_

b. _Have immature lung RDS._

372   10. Baby Marcia was considered to be born 2 weeks postterm. List three signs of post-maturity that you would look for.

a. _Dry parchment-like skin_

b. _long finger nails._

c. _Wide eyed alert expression_

Preterm infants receiving care for the crisis or complications of respiratory distress syndrome (RDS) represent a high percentage of the patients found in an NICU. Many of these newborns are transported considerable distances for treatment. Four-hour-old Wendy Hill is a 2-lb 15-oz (1332 g) infant with an estimated gestational age (EGA) of 30 weeks who has been admitted to the NICU this morning.

363   11. Her father arrives for the first time and asks to see his daughter. What kinds of information should be given him? What should he be encouraged to do? (Four items.)

a. _To touch and handle the child_

b. _Telephone number of NICU should be g_

c. _Taught how to gown_

d. _Tell about procedures before doing them_

- Assure them that most NICU patient suffer no permanent disability

367

12. List four signs or clinical measurements you might observe that possibly would indicate the development of RDS.

    a. _Nasal flaring_

    b. _Grunting on respiration_

    c. _Increase retractions_

    d. _Increase respiratory rate (over 45 per_

368

13. Wendy's condition worsens, and she requires intubation and continuous positive airway pressure (CPAP) of 12 cm. Her father has been told by the physician why this is necessary, but later he asks the nurse for an explanation again. What can she say to help him understand about the tube, the CPAP setup, and its purpose?

368

14. Why is Wendy receiving antibiotics even though she does not have any infection?

    Because she is maintained on ventillation which predispose her to infection

366

15. Wendy has an indwelling arterial catheter. Identify two problems associated with umbilical catheterization that the nurse may be able to help prevent or detect.

    a. _Emboli, Sepsis_

    b. _hemmorahge_

362

16. The most frequently encountered medical problem in the NICU is:
    a. Prematurity
    b. Birth defects
    c. Perinatal asphyxia
    d. Jaundice

362

17. Ideally, the facility that provides the NICU also should have a:
    a. High-risk obstetric department
    b. Medical intensive care unit
    c. Rehabilitation unit
    d. Cardiac intensive care unit

363

18. The nurse-patient ratio for critically ill infants or those coming immediately from surgery usually is:
    a. 1:1
    b. 1:2
    c. 2:1
    d. 2:3

363   19. Before and after handling any infant or piece of equipment involved in his or her care, nursery personnel must:
    a. Scrub hands with a brush
    b. Meticulously wash hands
    c. Wear a mask
    d. Put on a cover gown

368   20. Current treatment of RDS (until other forms of treatment are more available) is aimed at supporting the infant by assisting his oxygenation and ventilation until the lungs begin to produce surfactant, usually after:
    a. 12 hours
    b. 2 or 3 days
    c. 1 week
    d. About 10 days

368   21. The purpose of CPAP includes all of the following EXCEPT:
    a. Preventing atelectasis
    b. Improving oxygenation
    c. Decreasing the work of breathing
    d. Elevating body temperature

368   22. Infants receiving increased pressure therapy (by CPAP or mechanical ventilators) are at risk for all of the following complications except:
    a. Pneumothorax
    b. Infection
    c. Cardiovascular disturbances
    d. Hypovolemic shock

370   23. Cytomegalovirus (CMV) is the most common intrauterine infection known. Infants with CMV are usually:
    a. Hypoglycemic
    b. Septic
    c. Postmature
    d. Microcephalic

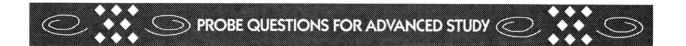

PROBE QUESTIONS FOR ADVANCED STUDY

1. The shock and heartbreak of sudden infant death syndrome (SIDS) is an overwhelming tragedy that leaves parents with devastating feelings and emotions. What are some of the common findings in cases with SIDS? What does the current research seem to indicate regarding the nature of this condition? How important is the position of the infant during sleep? Discuss the role of the nurse in providing support to the parents of SIDS victims.

REFERENCES

American Academy of Pediatrics: Positioning and SIDS, *Pediatrics* 89(6):1120-1126, 1992.

Back, KJ: Sudden, unexpected pediatric death: caring for the parents, *Pediatr Nursing* 17(6):571-575, 1991.

Carlson JA: The psychologic effects of sudden infant death syndrome on parents, *J Pediatr Health Care* 7(3):77-88, 1993.

Hass JE et al: Relationship between epidemiologic risk factors and clinicopathologic findings in the sudden infant death syndrome, *Pediatrics* 91(1):106-112, 1993.

Kahn A et al: Prone or supine body position and sleep characteristics in infants, *Pediatrics* 91(6):1112-1115, 1993.

Lerner H: Sleep position of infants: applying research to practice, *MCN* 19:(5):275-277, 1993.

2. A small infant was born after a 33-week pregnancy that was complicated by hemorrhage. Urine screen after birth was positive for cocaine. Cocaine is cleared from adult urine in approximately 24 hours. How long does cocaine persist in the urine of neonates? List the symptoms of cocaine exposure in the newborn. Discuss the neurobehavioral profiles of neonates exposed to cocaine before birth. How widespread is the abuse of cocaine among pregnant women?

REFERENCES

Forrest DC: The cocaine-exposed infant Part I identification and assessment, *J Pediatr Health Care* 8(1):3-6, 1994.

Forrest DC: The cocaine-exposed infant Part II intervention and teaching, *J Pediatr Health Care* 8(1):7-11, 1994.

Mayes LC et al: Neurobehavioral profiles of neonates exposed to cocaine prenatally, *Pediatrics* 91(4):778-783, 1993.

3. Meeting the nutritional needs of the premature infant who has been discharged from the NICU can be difficult. Breast-feeding is considered optimum for newborns but may not be possible for the premature infant. What determines the infant's formula needs? What percent of the caloric intake does the low-birth-weight infant use for basal metabolism? Define growth failure and discuss how gastrointestinal impairment affects growth.

REFERENCES

Gardner SL and Hagedirb MI: Physiologic sequelae of prematurity: the nurse practitioner's role. Part V. Feeding difficulties and growth failure, *J Pediatr Health Care* 5(3):122-134, 1991.

Pinyerd BJ: Assessment of infant growth, *J Pediatr Health Care* 6(5-part 2):302-308, 1992.

Snow SS and Fry ME: Formula feeding in the first year of life, *Pediatr Nursing* 16(5):442-446, 1990.

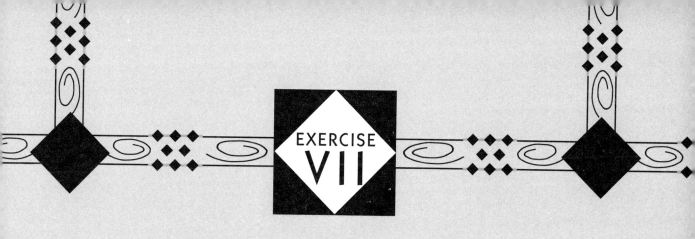

DEVELOPMENTAL
HEALTH
PROMOTION

Every nurse interested in the care of children needs a basic understanding of genetics, as well as human growth and development. In caring for children, the nurse must have an awareness of the approximate ages at which the child is capable of various activities and functions and which different types of behavior are likely to emerge. The nurse needs to know that there are genetic and environmental influences and limitation on growth and development, and he or she must realize that preventive pediatrics, which includes counseling parents, is a very important aspect of pediatric nursing. Knowledge of nutrition, immunization, and child safety will assist the nurse in fostering the child's growth and development while caring for a client in illness and in health. Chapters 20, 21, 22, and 23 provide information that will help the student deliver preventive health care to children and their parents.

CLINICAL TIE-IN

1. How does the pediatric unit differ from units that have adult patients?

2. Look at the Kardex and note the various illnesses listed. How do they differ from adult illnesses? Could any of these illnesses be prevented?
3. Can a little child tell you why he or she is in the hospital? What implications does this have for the pediatric nurse?
4. Young children will usually eat better in a group. Is there a dining place on the unit where children can eat together?
5. Check your patient's immunization record. Is it up to date? What resources are available in your community for immunizations?
6. During the past 2 weeks how many children have been admitted to the hospital because of injuries? What kinds of problems were encountered? How could they have been avoided?
7. Where is the nearest poison control center? To whom will the center give information?

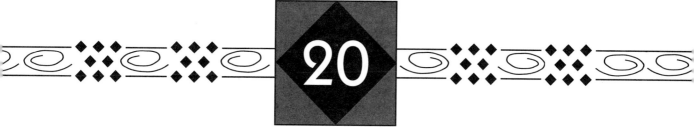

Genetic and Environmental Factors

Page Reference

1. Define the following terms.

380   a. Growth _Increase in structure_

380   b. Development _Increase in function_

380   c. Maturation _the inherited tendencies begin to unfold independent of any special practice or training_

381   d. Genes _Elements of defined lengths of DNA_

382   e. Pedigree _Construction of a chart that use standard symbols to designate family members_

382   f. Chromosomes _Microscopic structures within the nucleus of a cell that contain a species_

155

380

2. The terms growth and development often appear together and at times seem to be used as synonyms. However, they actually refer to different concepts. From your recent nursing experience, identify by first name and describe a patient who:
    a. Demonstrates normal growth but retarded development

    Certain type of mental retardation
    Down Syndrome.

    b. Demonstrates normal development but delayed growth

    End stage Renal disease
    Chronic heart disease
    Diabetes

381

3. State five principles of growth and development.
    a. In Sequence - They occur in orderly sequence.
    b. Continuity - although continuous they have period of lull & spurt.
    c. At it own rate - Highly individualize rate from child to child.
    d. All parts and function does not mature at the same time (might be advance in reading slow in
    e. Grow & Develop as a whole, socially, emotionally Spiritual being

380

4. Jimmy (5 years old) and John (12 months old) are brothers. Jimmy sat a 6 months and walked at 9 months. John sat at 9 months, can now stand alone, but cannot walk. His worried mother asks you if something is wrong with John because he is "so slow." How will you reply to this mother?

    Each child grow at its own rate

381-386

5. List the two main types of influences that can either inhibit or enhance growth and development. Give examples of each.

a. _Enviroment - Inhibit - poor nutrition_
enhance - (good nutrition

b. _Genetic - Inhibit - Cyctic Fibrosis, sickle_
cell disease Enhance - Early detection PKU

381-386

6. Genes, the elements of inheritance, are defined lengths of

381   a. _DNA_ found in the

381   b. _chromosomes_ within the nucleus of each cell. Each normal human

being has _46 chromosomes_

381   c. _46_ chromosomes in his body cells.

381   d. _23_ of these chromosomes were donated by his mother, the other

381   e. _23_ by his father. The two chromosomes X and Y, which determine the sex of the individual, are called sex chromosomes. All other chromosomes are called

382   f. _autosomes_ . An orderly arrangement of an individual's autosomal and sex chromosomes according to size, shape, and banding pattern as they appear in cutouts of photographic enlargements is known as a

382   g. _Karyotype_ . Chromosomal abnormalities result from

385   h. _various failures in the produce of ova_
and sperm with two gonads (meosis
and

385   i. _motosis, abnormal sperm tun of_
egs

382

7. The genes found in the chromosomes exist in pairs. A dominant gene will be expressed regardless of the complementary gene contributed by the other parent.

a. In the space below depict the possible genetic outcome of the mating of a woman having genetically dominant neurofibromatosis (Dn) with a man who does not carry this trait (nn). Each time she conceives a child she has what per

centage chance of carrying the gene of this disease? _50 %_

	Affected mother Dn	**Normal father** nn
	Dn	nn
X	Dn x	nn x
Y	DN y	nn y

382

b. Is the affected parent homozygous or heterozygous for the dominant trait?

_____ heterozygous _____

386

c. Name one other disease that is classified as dominant.

_____ dwarfism _____

8. Certain genes are recessive rather than dominant.

382-383

a. If a cystic fibrosis carrier marries another cystic fibrosis carrier, each child have

what percentage of being born with this serious disease? ___ 25 % ___
Work out this genetic problem.

Carrier mother
Nr

Carrier father
Nr

25 % carrier
50 % don't

382
386

b. Are these parents homozygous or heterozygous for the trait? ___ homozygous ___

c. Name two other diseases that are classified as recessive.

(1) ___ Sickle cell ___

(2) ___ albinism ___

384

9. a. X-linked recessive genetic disorders can be inherited in what manner?

mother making her daughter carrier and
50 % son the disease found X linked chromos

384

b. Work out this genetic problem.

Carrier mother
Xx

Carrier father
xy

386   c. Name two other diseases that are classified as X-linked recessive.

    (1) _Hemophilia_____

    (2) _Muscular Dystrophy_____

386   10. What is the purpose of the Human Genome Project?

Creating a complete map and sequence of all three billion base pairs of DNA that make up human genetic complement.

386   11. What is the ultimate goal of the Human Genome Project?

Better understanding of genetic disease in general

386   12. Amniocentesis usually is performed at a gestational age of ___16 weeks__

386   13. Is there any other method used for prenatal diagnosis other than amniocentesis? Explain.

chronic villa sampling. — an alternative prenatal approach diagnosis

Transcervical & trans.

389   14. The primary use of growth charts is to detect clinical disturbances in growth and

nutrition_____

15. John (10 years old) has eight second teeth. His new teeth are stained.

391-392 a. Should John have more permanent teeth at his age? _____ no _____.

391 b. What might have caused the dental staining? __ Is mother taking the antibiotic tetracycline before he was born or taken by John before he was eight years old.

393 16. Effective use of hands to grasp and manipulate objects is an important skill shared by only a few creatures on our plant. According to Gesell, prehension usually follows a certain pattern. Add five more stages and samples of behavior to the pattern below.

Stage	Sample behavior
Example: 12 weeks	Looks at cube
a. 20 weeks.	looks and approaches
b. 24 weeks	" crudely grasps with whole ha
c. 36 weeks.	" and deftly grasp ī fingers
d. 52 weeks.	looks grasps with forefingers thumb & deftl
e. 15 months	looks grasps and releases build a tower of blocks

394 17. The following are familiar guideposts in the motor development of an infant. Indicate on the bar the average age range of their appearance.
a. Lifts chest and head
b. Sits up with support
c. Sits up alone, steadily, without support
d. Creeps
e. Stands holding onto support
f. Stands alone, walks with help
g. Walks alone

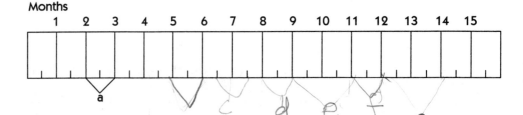

Months
1 2 3 4 5 6 7 8 9 10 11 12 13 14 15

Jane, 5 years old, had her tonsils removed 2 weeks ago. Her mother relates that Jane has had "just one sore throat after another." Jane is 41 inches tall and weighs 34 lb. At birth she weighed 7 lb 9 $^1/_2$ oz and measured 20 inches. The mother has been told by Jane's physician that both her sisters, ages 3 and 8 years, are in the 90th percentile for weight and height for children of their ages. She wants to know Jane's percentile and her prospects for growth.

388-389   18. What does a percentile rank of 90 mean?

19. Plot the percentile rank of Jane on the anthropometric chart (See Appendix E, p. 877).

388-389   20. How would you interpret Jane's growth prospects to her mother?

386   21. Which of the following conditions is the result of a numeric disorder of the sex chromosomes?
a. Down syndrome
b. Marfan's syndrome
c. Aldrich syndrome
d. Turner's syndrome

384, 386   22. Which of the following conditions is thought to be the result of a combination of genetic differences or defects and environmental factors?
a. Anencephaly
b. Hemophilia A
c. Phenylketonuria
d. Cystic fibrosis

382   23. An alteration in an individual's genetic makeup that might be inherited by his children is called a:
       a. Pedigree
       b. Mosaic
       c. Karyotype
       d. Mutation

382   24. The mendelian disorders can be subdivided into how many distinct patterns of inheritance?
       a. 2
       b. 3
       c. 4
       d. 5

385   25. One kind of chromosome change that can be inherited involves the transfer of material between two chromosomes and is called a:
       a. Nondisjunction
       b. Mosaicism
       c. Mutation
       d. Translocation

386   26. Down syndrome (Trisomy 23), which produces mental retardation and other physical deviations, is most often the result of:
       a. Advanced paternal age
       b. Autosomal dominant inheritance
       c. Advanced maternal age
       d. Autosomal recessive inheritance

386   27. Multifactorial disorders are the result of an interaction between multiple defective genes and the environment. Which one of the following conditions is an example of this disorder?
       a. Phenylketonuria
       b. Turner's syndrome
       c. Pyloric stenosis
       d. Hurler's syndrome

386   28. In which one of the following disorders will an affected female's offspring have a 50% chance of being affected?
       a. Vitamin D-resistant rickets
       b. Tay-Sachs disease
       c. Spina bifida
       d. Klinefelter's syndrome

386   29. A reduction of the total number of autosomal chromosomes is:
       a. Not compatible with life
       b. The result of consanguinity
       c. Compatible with life
       d. Homozygous for males

389   30. The newborn head constitutes about:
       a. One third the total body length
       b. One fourth the total body length
       c. One eighth the total body length
       d. One tenth the total body length

389   31. Cartilage gradually is replaced by bone; this process is called:
        a. Ossification
        b. Prehension
        c. Maturation
        d. Resorption

388   32. The best method of evaluating a child's general growth progress is by comparing
        the child from time to time with:
        a. Himself
        b. Siblings
        c. Peers
        d. Parents

398   33. In all cultures the principal provider of nurture to the child is the:
        a. Family
        b. Father
        c. Mother
        d. Parents

399-400 34. Parenting is most likely to be learned:
        a. During the early school years
        b. Through role modeling of parents
        c. During the early adolescent years
        d. Through books featuring homemaking

399   35. Of the following styles of parenting, which is likely to be the most effective in that
        it seeks input from both the child and the parent in problem solving and encour-
        ages analysis and self-discipline?
        a. Authoritarian
        b. Permissive
        c. Autocratic
        d. Authoritative

399   36. Which style of parenting emphasizes "obedience and respect of parental role?"
        a. Authoritative
        b. Permissive
        c. Democratic
        d. Autocratic

399   37. Which one of the following factors is necessary for any relationship to endure?
        a. Communication
        b. Self-respect
        c. Common sense
        d. Education

400   38. A supportive communication technique that reflects back to the child and his feel-
        ings is:
        a. Active-listening
        b. Acknowledgement responses
        c. Passive listening
        d. Silent behavior

401   39. Which one of the following techniques used to shape behavior is least acceptable in society today?
          a. Teaching by example
          b. Corporal punishment
          c. Active listening
          d. Employing "time out"

401   40. Which of the following has the most significant influence on the development of a child's basic moral and spiritual concepts?
          a. The church
          b. The school
          c. The community
          d. The home

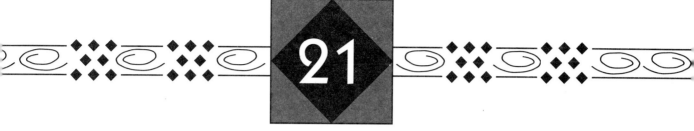

Developmental Assessment

Page Reference

1. Fill in the missing data in the following progression of growth and development.

404   a. A newborn usually gains approximately <u>5-7 oz</u> each week.

407   b. Birth weight doubles at <u>5 month</u> .

412   c. Birth weight triples at <u>1 year 12 month</u>

412   d. Average height increases <u>10 inches</u> during the first year.

415   e. Average height increases <u>5 inches</u> during the second year.

429   f. Growth in height speeds up again at ages <u>10</u> to <u>14</u> for girls and <u>12</u> to <u>16</u> in boys.

409   g. An infant begins to recognize and avoid strangers at <u>7 - 9 months</u>.

409   h. The first primary toot erupts at <u>6</u> . It usually is located at <u>2 lower incisors</u>.

415   i. Bowel control may be achieved by <u>24</u> months.

417   j. Daytime bladder control may be achieved by <u>3</u> years.

433   2. For what purpose is the Denver II Screening Test administered?

<u>To detect any problem is developent</u>

409   3. The baby's progress on all fours, trunk supported by the floor, is called:
     a. Cruising   c. Creeping
     b. Crawling   d. Hitching

411   4. An infant can move forward with trunk above floor by age:
     a. 5 months   c. 9 months
     b. 7 months   d. 12 months

409   5. An infant vocalizes ma-ma or da-da at about:
a. 3 months   c. 10 months
b. 5 months   d. 12 months

408   6. An infant usually is able to hold a rattle by:
a. 1 month   c. 3 months
b. 2 months   d. 4 months

413   7. Most children have a vocabulary of 6 to 18 words and can follow simple commands by age:
a. 9-12 months   c. 15-18 months
b. 12-15 months   d. 18-20 months

433   8. The Denver II Screening Test evaluates children to age:
a. 3 years   c. 5 years
b. 4 years   d. 6 years

404   9. During the first 6 months the infant usually gains:
a. 1 oz/day   c. 1 lb/month
b. 1 lb/week   d. 2 lb/month

407   10. Healthy infants usually understand and respond to their name at age:
a. 1 month   c. 5 months
b. 3 months   d. 12 months

405   11. The posterior fontanel may close as early as:
a. 1 month   c. 3 months
b. 2 months   d. 4 months

407   12. The schedule for introduction of semisolid foods depends on the infant and the physician. However, most infants are offered cereal at:
a. 1 to 2 months   c. 5 to 6 months
b. 3 to 4 months   d. 7 to 8 months

407   13. The Moro reflex should be absent by age:
a. 1 month   c. 4 months
b. 2 months   d. 6 months

413   14. The anterior fontanel normally closes by:
a. 6 months   c. 18 months
b. 12 months   d. 21 months

415   15. Bowel control may be achieved by age:
a. 12 months   c. 24 months
b. 18 months   d. 36 months

416   16. The child has a complete set of primary teeth at age:
a. 12 months   c. 30 months
b. 24 months   d. 36 months

423   17. The first permanent teeth erupt at age:
a. 4 years   c. 6 years
b. 5 years   d. 8 years

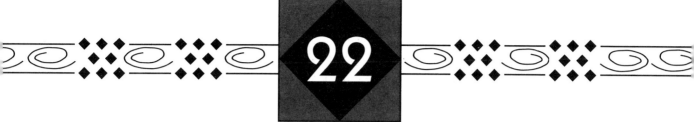

Child Health
Promotion

Page Reference

1. Health supervision can be carried out by the private physician, the nurse practitioner, a public facility, or a child health conference.

439 a. Identify at least three components of health supervision and "well child care."

(1) _Promote health_

(2) _Prevent disease_

(3) _Provide anticipatory guidance for development_ & parenting issues

439-440 b. How often should a child be evaluated during the early years of life?

1. within 1 week of birth
2. monthly for 6 months
3. every other month until first birthday.
3. 2-4 visits during second year.
4. after 3 years should be annually.

440 c. When should dental supervision begin? ① Before any apparent problem

② Before the childs 3rd birthday

446

2. All body systems and tissues depend on proper nourishment for their growth and maintenance.
   a. What three functions within the body must food perform?
      (1) Provide heat & energy.
      (2) Build & repair body tissues.
      (3) Regulate body processes
   b. List the eight basic substances that are essential to body processes.
      (1) Oxygen
      (2) water.
      (3) Protein
      (4) Carbohydrates
      (5) fats.
      (6) Minerals
      (7) Vitiamins
      (8) fibers

446

3. To keep pace with normal fluid losses, how much fluid must the infant receive daily? An equal fluid intake 100 ml/100 kilocal

447

4. What is meant by the phrase essential amino acids? _____

447

5. What is meant by the term complete and incomplete proteins? Give two examples of each.
   Complete proteins contain essential amino ac
   eg: poultry, fish meat, eggs.

   Incomplete proteins cantain many amino acid
   but not all essential ones.
   eg: vegetables & grains

451

6. Two vitamins that may be stored and become excessive in the body are:
   a. Vitamin A
   b. D

451   7. The four fat-soluble vitamins are:

a. _A_

b. _D_

c.. _E_

d.. _K_

449   8. Two minerals most likely to be deficient in a child's diet are:

a. _Iron_

b. _Calcium_

447   9. Define calorie as used in planning diets. _The amount of heat needed to raise the temperature of 1 kilogram of water 1°_

447   10. What are the caloric values for the following energy-producing food elements?

a. Carbohydrates   _4_ calories/g

b. Proteins   _4_ calories/g

c. Fats   _9_ calories/g

442   11. At what age does the protrusion reflex disappear? _4 months_

443   12. Self-feeding:

a. At what age do babies begin to feed themselves? _Skills develop at 6 months. at 7 months hold bottle. 8-5 months feed self crackers._

b. At what age is self-feeding accomplished? _12-18 month_

13. A person is able to build up defenses against certain infectious diseases through immunization.

456
454   a. At what age should immunization begin? _Hepatitis B is given at birth before discharge_

b. List seven common childhood diseases that can be prevented through immunization.

(1) _mumps_

(2) _Polio_

(3) _measles_

(4) _tentanus_

(5) _Hepatitis B_

(6) _rubella_

(7) _Diptheria_

453

    c. Recommendations for immunizing infants and children are governed by whom?

        Advisory Committee on Immunization Practices of US Public Serice

458

    d. Give three instances when immunization procedures are contraindicated.

        (1) *Anaphylactic - like reactions*

        (2) *Moderate - or severe illness with or without fever*

        (3) *DTP or DTAP should not be repeated if encephalop*

453

    e. Passive immunity acquired from the infant's mother usually persists for

        4 - 6 month

453

    f. What is the difference between passive and active immunity?

        Passive immunity is antigen given, eg. shot

        Active immunity - formation of antigens by patient himself.

463

14. The greatest threat to the health and well being of the child today is injury. List five factors associated with childhood injuries.

    a. *Age of child*

    b. *Gender of Child*

    c. *Non white child has higher incidents of accidents*

    d. *Most injuries occur during spring & summer*

    90% e. *High injuries happen at home.*

467

15. The greatest number of childhood poisonings occurs in children under 4 years of age.

    a. Why is this so? *Its the age of Curlosity. Children are not selective about what they ingest*

470

    b. List five suggestions you can give to parents that can help prevent accidental poisoning.

    (1) *Household products & medicine should be kept out of the reach child*

    (2) *All products should be properly label.*

    use correct name

    (3) *Medicine should never be referred to as candy*

    (4) *a light should be turn on when one is giving or taki*

    (5) *Medicine cabinet should be cleaned out periodically.*

467

c. It is most important to empty the child's stomach when he has ingested a potential poison. However, emesis should not be induced in some instances. List three.

(1) _Corrosives — lye or strong acid_

(2) child unconcious
(3) child convalescing

(2) _hydrocarbons —) kerosene, gasoline._

(3) _Strychnine — : fuel oil, paint thinner_

467

d. Every parent of a toddler should have a bottle of syrup of ipecac in the home. Why? What dose should be used?

Use to induce emesis in case of i positin,
~ 15 mL followed by glass of water'

439

16. Child Health supervision is designed to provide all of the following *EXCEPT*:
    a. Provide developmental guidance
    b. Help with childrearing counseling
    c. Protect against certain preventable diseases
    d. Provide funds for needy families

440

17. The American Academy of Pediatrics urges that all bottle-fed infants be given an iron-fortified formula during the first:
    a. 3 months
    b. 6 months
    c. 9 months
    d. 12 months

442

18. Skim milk is inadequate in fat, fatty acid, and calories. It also has four times the estimated requirement of protein needed by the infant. Therefore it should not be given to young children before age:
    a. 1 year
    b. 2 years
    c. 3 years
    d. 4 years

450

19. Vitamin A deficiency can lead to:
    a. Anemia
    b. Night blindness
    c. Rickets
    d. Scurvy

450

20. Vitamin C deficiency can manifest itself as:
    a. Nausea and vomiting
    b. Loose teeth and slow growth
    c. Photophobia and cataracts
    d. Ulcers and fissures of the tongue

449   21. If community water is not sufficiently fluoridated naturally, supplemental fluoride should be prescribed and given from birth until the eruption of:
        a. All primary teeth
        b. The first molars
        c. All permanent teeth
        d. The second molars

446   22. Amino acids are used for all of the following *EXCEPT*:
        a. Tissue growth and repair
        b. Construction of antibodies and hormones
        c. Prevention of tooth decay and staining
        d. Heat and energy

443   23. New foods should be offered when the baby is hungry and:
        a. After his formula
        b. Before his formula
        c. At night
        d. In the morning

448   24. Which of the following minerals is essential for normal heart action and blood clotting?
        a. Potassium
        b. Calcium
        c. Iron
        d. Sodium

449   25. The greatest incidence of iron-deficiency anemia occurs in:
        a. Adolescent boys
        b. Infants and young children
        c. School-age children
        d. Preschool boys and girls

454   26. The recommended schedule for active immunization during the first 6 months includes diphtheria-tetanus-pertussis, Haemophilus type b conjugate, hepatitis B and:
        a. Measles vaccine
        b. Oral poliovirus
        c. Rubella vaccine
        d. Mumps vaccine

461   27. Immune globulin confers temporary immunity that is attained in approximately 2 days and last from:
        a. 1 week to 1 month
        b. 1 to 6 weeks
        c. 4 weeks to 2 months
        d. 6 weeks to 6 months

461   28. Immune globulin has been clearly documented to be helpful in preventing antibody deficiency disease and:
        a. Measles and pancreatitis
        b. Measles and chickenpox
        c. Measles and infectious hepatitis (HAV)
        d. Measles and rubella

459 29. Routine immunization against smallpox is no longer recommended because:
   a. Children now have natural immunity against smallpox
   b. The risk of complications outweighs the risk of acquiring the disease
   c. The disease has been eradicated
   d. The vaccine is no longer effective

459 30. *Haemophilus* type b conjugate vaccine is routinely recommended for all young children. Which one of the following conditions is *least likely* to present an increased risk of *H. influenzae* infections in children?
   a. Day-care facilities
   b. Sickle cell disease
   c. Certain chronic illnesses
   d. School-age populations

463 31. Of the following, the one true statement is that:
   a. Boys at all ages have fewer injuries than girls
   b. The nonwhite population has a low incidence of injuries
   c. A higher percentage of injuries occurs outside the home
   d. Toddlers are most vulnerable to injuries

465 32. Fundamental prerequisites of injury prevention for school-age children are:
   a. Education, discipline, and obedience
   b. Courage, good balance, and proper equipment
   c. A safe environment and constant supervision
   d. A sense of self-worth and accomplishment

467 33. The majority of childhood poisonings are preventable. Most poisonings occur:
   a. In the parent's garage
   b. In the family house
   c. In the neighbor's house
   d. In the grandparent's house

467 34. The majority of poisonings occur in children under:
   a. 1 year
   b. 4 years
   c. 10 years
   d. 15 years

467 35. Removal is the most important aspect of poison management. However, emesis should *not* be induced if the ingested substance is:
   a. Strychnine
   b. Diazepam (Valium)
   c. Aspirin
   d. Acetaminophen (Tylenol)

471 36. A powerful physical antidote that adsorbs most poisons is:
   a. Dimercaprol (BAL)
   b. Activated charcoal
   c. Syrup of ipecac
   d. Apomorphine

471   37. In cases of acute salicylate poisoning in children, the first manifestation is:
a. Fever
b. Hyperpnea
c. Bleeding
d. Tremor

471   38. The immediate treatment of acute salicylate poisoning is:
a. Gastric lavage
b. Induced emesis
c. Cool sponging
d. Blood transfusions

472   39. Neglected, nonaccidentally injured children are typically under age:
a. 1 year
b. 2 years
c. 3 years
d. 5 years

472   40. As part of public child welfare services, most communities have established protective services for neglected and abused children. A protective service exists to accomplish all the tasks below *EXCEPT*:
a. Providing follow-up supervision of abused children
b. Helping parents who want help
c. Punishing parents who abuse their children
d. Protecting children from abuse

STUDENT'S NAME _____

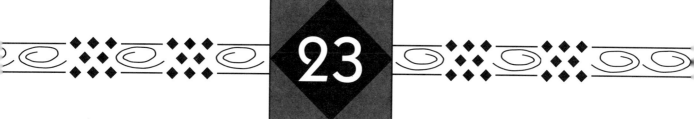

Laboratory Screening in Child Health

Page Reference

490-491

1. Blood specimens usually are secured by the physician or laboratory personnel. What is the nurse's responsibility during the collection of specimens?

   _____

   _____

2. Complete the following information.

   Normal values for newborn and young children

   a. *Blood*

482   RBC   _____

482   WBC   _____

481   Hematocrit   _____

481   Hemoglobin   _____

   b. *Urine*

493   Color   _____

492   Acetone   _____

492   Albumin   _____

492   Glucose   _____   _____

493   Cells   _____

493   Casts   _____

493   Specific gravity   _____

494   pH   _____

175

499
3. What is the routine preparation for a barium enema in the hospital pediatric unit where you are assigned?

500
4. What is the routine preparation for a gastrointestinal x-ray film series in young children?

497-498
5. Match the appropriate items involving diagnostic tests and their use.

_____ Cystic fibrosis

_____ Abnormalities in electric impulses of the heart

_____ Prenatal lung maturity

_____ Meningitis

_____ Abnormalities of the brain waves

a. Lecithin/sphingomyelin (L/S) ratio
b. Lumbar puncture
c. Electrocardiogram (ECG, EKG)
d. Sweat test
e. Electroencephalogram (EEG)

482
6. A test that identifies microorganisms circulating in the bloodstream is:
a. WBC differential
b. Antistreptolysin O titer
c. RBC count
d. Blood culture

484
7. A test that helps determine kidney disease or urinary obstruction is:
a. Blood urea nitrogen
b. Blood glucose
c. C-reactive protein
d. Specific gravity

496
8. A test that detects the presence of blood in the feces is:
a. RBC count
b. Addis count
c. Occult blood
d. Hematocrit

477   9. Although the nurse does not need to know the details of all diagnostic tests, she should know all of the following information regarding any specific test *EXCEPT*:
            a. The purpose
            b. Patient preparation
            c. Exact cost
            d. Follow-up care

478   10. Laboratory procedures differ in various hospitals. Thus, before participation in any test, the nurse should consult the:
            a. Physician
            b. Laboratory technician
            c. Team leader
            d. Procedure manual

478   11. Which one of the following is not an appropriate venipuncture site?
            a. Jugular vein
            b. Ankle vein
            c. Arm vein
            d. Femoral vein

485   12. Which one of the following blood tests requires the patient to fast?
            a. Rh factor
            b. Coombs test
            c. Glucose tolerance
            d. Hematocrit

483   13. Which one of the four main blood types found in the general population is most common?
            a. A
            b. B
            c. AB
            d. O

485   14. All newborn infants are required to be screened for hypothyroidism and:
            a. Phenylketonuria
            b. Neuroblastoma
            c. Fetal lung maturity
            d. Cystic fibrosis

500   15. Which one of the following tests provides a visual display of abnormal tissue within the skull and is useful in diagnosing brain tumors?
            a. Computerized transaxial tomography
            b. Pneumoencephalogram
            c. Ventriculogram
            d. Electroencephalogram

1. Child abuse (nonaccidental injury) cases continue to rise. How widespread and serious are child abuse and child sexual abuse in the United States? What is the leading cause of death from nonaccidental injury? Is abuse a premeditated behavior? How can you recognize abuse in the young child? What is the nurse's primary concern when caring for a child who has been abused?

REFERENCES

Chadwick DL: The diagnosis of inflicted injury on infants and young children, *Pediatr Annals* 21(8):477-483, 1992.

Devlin BK and Reynolds E: Child abuse: how to recognize it, how to intervene, *Am J Nurs* 94(3):26-31, 1994.

Finkelhor D: Epidemiological factors in the clinical identification of child sexual abuse, *Child Abuse Neglect* 17(1):67-70, 1993.

Hyden PW and Gallagher TA: Child abuse intervention in the emergency room, *Pediatr Clin North Am* 39(5):1053-1081, 1992.

2. Drowning ranks second as the leading cause of death in young children. Every year a significant number of children experience near drowning and suffer irreversible brain injury. Define near-drowning (nonfatal submersion). Discuss the prognosis of near-drowning in children who remain comatose 24 hours after submersion. How can nurses assist the family in planning for the care of a disabled child at home?

REFERENCES

Batton SL, Jardine DS, and Morray JP: Serial neurologic examinations after near drowning and outcome, *Arch Pediatr Adolescent Med* 148(2):167-170, 1994.

Coffman SP: Home care of the child and family after near drowning, *J Pediatr Health Care* 6(1):18-24, 1992.

Norris MKG: Action STAT! Pediatric near drowning, *Nursing* 23(5):33, 1993.

3. How do personal values relate to the likelihood of participating in high-risk sexual behaviors? Why are adolescents at high risk for acquired immunodeficiency syndrome (AIDS)? Presently, teaching people how to avoid becoming infected with the human immunodeficiency virus is the only strategy for reducing the spread of AIDS. Discuss how nurses can be successful in teaching AIDS prevention to adolescents. Discuss the drug therapy currently available for the health maintenance of AIDS patients.

REFERENCES

Jemmott LS: AIDS risk among black male adolescents: implications for nursing interventions, *J Pediatr Health Care* 7(1):3-11, 1993.

Rozmus CL and Edgil AE: Values, knowledge, and attitudes about acquired immunodeficiency syndrome in rural adolescents, *J Pediatr Health Care* 7(4):167-173, 1993.

Sagraves R: Drug therapy for human immunodeficiency virus infection in children, *J Pediatr Health Care* 7(4):177-184, 1993.

4. Inattention, impulsivity, and hyperactivity are behaviors characteristic of a syndrome called Attention Deficit Hyperactivity Disorder (ADHD). About 4% to 5% of all elementary children are said to have this disorder. Describe the behavior of the child who has this disorder, both in the home and school environments. How is ADHD evaluated? Discuss some of the therapeutic modalities (behavioral, psychodynamic, and pharmacological) and the follow-up care of children with ADHD.

REFERENCES

Comfort RL: Living with an unconventional child, *J Pediatr Health Care* 6(3):114-120, 1992.

Long N, Rickert VI, Ashcraft EW: Bibliotherapy as an adjunct to stimulant medication in the treatment of attention-deficit hyperactivity disorder, *J Pediatr Health Care* 7(2):82-88, 1993.

Murphy MA, Hagerman RJ: Attention deficit hyperactivity disorder in children: diagnosis, treatment, and follow-up, *J Pediatr Health Care* 6(1):2-11, 1992.

Smitherman CH: A drug to ease attention deficit-hyperactivity disorder, *Am J Maternal Child Nursing* 15(6):362-365, 1990.

5. One often gains considerable information by studying in greater depth the growth and developmental patterns of one or more patients. Such a study can alert you to average differences in body size, physiology, and abilities that normally occur in children with the passage of time. It also should emphasize the effects of such factors as genetic heritage, nutrition, sensory stimulation, and illness of various types on the growth and development of the child. The information obtained assists you in determining the best approach to an individual child and occasionally offers diagnostic information to the physician. Usually the study has more learning value if the child selected for evaluation is from 6 months to 4 years of age. A suggested model follows.

a. Patient's initials, age, length of observation.

b. Family composition, approximate socioeconomic and educational backgrounds, and cultural heritage. Include evaluation of parent-child relationships and the parents' ability to cope.

c. Health history (previous illness or experiences that may affect growth and development).

d. Present illness (anatomical, physiological, and psychological problems associated with the diagnosis). The basic treatment plan.

e. Evaluation of developmental level as revealed by motor control, vocalization, socialization, and intellectual skills. Use three columns as shown below and expand as needed. Consult the Denver II Screening Test, as well as your text discussion, for detailed forms.

f. Have the child's growth and development been affected by the health history? How has the child responded to hospitalization? How have you tried to help the child adjust?

Characteristics	Norms for age	Patient's data and percentile rank	How did findings affect nursing care?*
Weight Height Head size (in children less than 1 year) Pulse ranges Respiration ranges Motor control Vocalization Socialization Nutrition (give a sample day's menu)			

*For example, type of equipment and clothing needed, safety precautions, kinds of procedures carried out, expectations, or methods of communication and assurance.

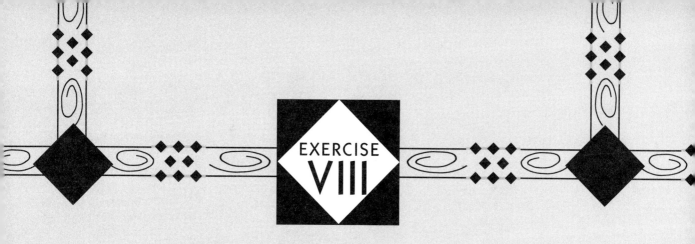

THE HOSPITALIZED CHILD AND FAMILY

In the past hospitalization was almost always traumatic, and in some cases the adverse effects were long lasting. Today a great deal is done to try to make hospitalization less fearful and less difficult. Often the parent makes a judgment about the hospital based on the nurses' behavior. If you are assigned to the important task of admission, you can help the parent-child unit by first recognizing both parent and child. Explain to the child what you are doing in a manner that the parent can hear too. When parents perceive the nurse as secure in his or her knowledge, warm and gentle, a trusting relationship begins and fears of hospitalization subside. Chapters 24, 25, 26, 27, and 28 provide information that will help the student deliver a high quality of nursing care to children and their parents.

CLINICAL TIE-IN

1. What information does the hospital ask on the questionnaire sent to the child and family before admission? How does the parent know in advance that an admission party is held on certain days?
2. Is there a play area in the hospital for children? Who supervises the play area? If there is a person to help with playtime, what educational preparation is required for the position?
3. Are parents allowed to remain with children during procedures such as dressing changes, lumbar punctures, or brain scans? What considerations influence the decision to exclude or include the parent during a procedure?
4. Why can securing an appropriate urine specimen be particularly difficult in pediatrics?
5. Why is the amount of blood drawn for analysis from infants especially significant?
6. What guidelines are used to evaluate postoperative pain in preverbal children?
7. Is there a pediatric respiratory therapist available to administer inhalation medications and chest PT, or is the nurse responsible for these treatments?

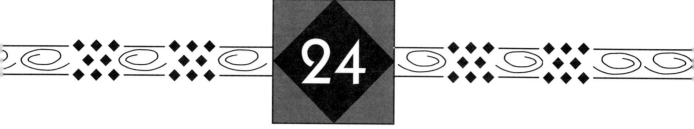

The Hospitalized Child

Page Reference

507

1. A child's reaction to illness and hospitalization is influenced by their parents' reactions and by their:

   a. Available support system.

   b. Developmental level.

   c. Previous experiences

510

2. What is meant by separation anxiety? What age group is most likely to be affected when hospitalized?

   When mother unable to come to the hospital for a prolong period and the child suffer from numerous traumatic factors.

   X When mother & child have healthy relationship

   Age 4

510

3. List the three phases of the "settling in" process as defined by Robertson, and briefly describe the child's behavior during each phase.

   a. Despair - Withdrawn

   b. Denial - accepting surrounding, suppressing feelings for parent

   c. Protest - child cry aloud, throwing self on floor

511

4. When might the effects of separation manifest themselves? After the child returns home

183

510   5. Mrs. Green must leave the hospital to go to work. How can you help her and her 3-year-old Tim, who is crying and begging her to stay?

Tell Mrs Green that the reason for him to be crying is because of the healthy reactions that they have established between her & her baby. Suggest she explain to the child in words that the child can under that she will be bac

507-509   6. List six different ways that many hospital pediatric departments, physicians, and nurses have tried to alter or improve their policies and procedures to reduce the trauma of hospitalization.

a. *Colorful booklets & pamphats*

b. *Telephone calls*

c. *Hospital tours*

d. *Pre admission orientation parties*

e. *Movies, Educational TV.*

f. *Puppet shows, Teaching dolls,*

507   7. Of the following persons, who is best able to prepare the child for hospitalization?
   a. Physician
   b. School nurse
   c. Parents ✓
   d. Friends

508   8. Which of the following should be the least important consideration when preparing a child for surgery?
   a. Age
   b. Developmental level
   c. Temperament
   d. Ethnicity ✓

508   9. One of the best guides to use when preparing a child for hospitalization is:
   a. Truthful assurance ✓
   b. Detailed explanations
   c. Complete information
   d. Surgical illustrations

512   10. Which one of the following nursing actions would be most helpful for Jimmy, age 4 years, who is to have an x-ray film taken at the bedside?
   a. Explain the procedure in advance ✓
   b. Wait until his parents come
   c. Explain the procedure to him after it is completed
   d. Show him some x-ray films

508   11. Which of the following is most helpful in preparing parents and children for hospitalization?
a. Coloring books
b. Puppet show
c. Tour of the hospital ✓
d. Telephone conversation

508   12. Which choice in the following listing would usually be most helpful in lessening a young child's distress during hospitalization?
a. Protecting the child from infection
b. Telling the child a story about animals
c. Showing the child how to call the nurse
d. Allowing the mother to bathe the child ✓

509   13. Which of the following would make it easier for the mother and father to continue their supportive role for hospitalized 1-year-old Mary?
a. Liberal visiting hours ✓
b. Conferences with the nursing staff
c. Books about her disease
d. A private room

508   14. Which of the following interventions is most helpful to the hospitalized child and to siblings?
a. Describing the pediatric services
b. Encouraging siblings to write
c. Allowing siblings to visit ✓
d. Reading about hospital experiences

509   15. The nurse can best encourage emotional growth of the hospitalized child by:
a. Accepting the child as he or she is ✓
b. Teaching good health habits
c. Making the child conform to the hospital's rules
d. Encouraging the child to stay in his or her own area

510   16. The risk involved with parent-child separation is greatest during:
a. Infancy
b. Toddlerhood ✓
c. Preschool
d. Adolescence

510   17. A mother is about to leave her 3-year-old child who is crying. Her most helpful parting comment would be:
a. "I'll be back; don't cry"
b. "Be good while I'm gone"
c. "I'll be back before suppertime" ✓
d. "I'll bring you a new toy"

511   18. Which of the following is most helpful in minimizing a 5-year-old child's anxiety during hospitalization?
a. The presence of supportive parents ✓
b. An opportunity to play each day
c. Freedom to ambulate about the ward
d. A supportive health care team

511   19. The school-age child is not so susceptible to separation anxiety if his or her illness is short. However, school-age children are most concerned and bothered by:
    a. Cost of hospitalization
    b. Loss of school days
    c. The disease process
    d. Loss of playmates

512   20. Whether hospitalization is ultimately a positive or negative experience for the adolescent depends to a large degree on:
    a. Sensitive care given by nurses
    b. Visitation of school friends
    c. Ability to participate in self care
    d. Collaboration with family members

512   21. Which of the following actions would be the *least traumatic* for a 5-year-old who has an order for an injection tomorrow?
    a. Telling the child that he or she will receive an injection tomorrow
    b. Waking the child from sleep to give the injection
    c. Telling the child about the injection just before giving it
    d. Giving the injection quickly while the child is sleeping

512   22. Which of the following nursing actions is considered to be *least important* for the school age child's emotional adjustment to an unpleasant procedure?
    a. An opportunity to talk about fears
    b. Answering the child's questions simply and honestly
    c. Telling how another child felt about the procedure
    d. Allowing the parent to explain the procedure

513   23. A common danger that can be avoided when a child is hospitalized over a long period of time is:
    a. Hostility
    b. Depression
    c. Aggression
    d. Dependency

513   24. The educational program for children in hospitals is the responsibility of the:
    a. Child's parents
    b. Child life worker
    c. Social worker
    d. Public school

513   25. A play program is designed for hospitalized children in an effort to protect the child from the effects of:
    a. Isolation
    b. Treatments
    c. Immobilization
    d. Depression

514   26. A healthy resolution of the negative aspects of the hospital experience may be lessened through:
    a. Exercise
    b. Education
    c. Play
    d. Reading

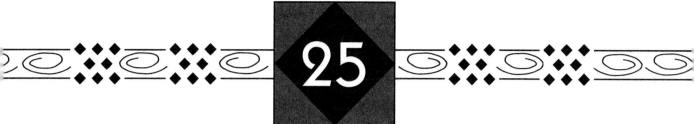

Hospital Admission and Discharge

Page Reference

517

1. Why is it necessary to check the child's weight and height during the admission procedure?

   To determine the dosage of medicine and general condition and progress

517

2. Children that must have their weight checked daily have what kind of problems? When is the weight check usually done?

   Diarrhea & vomiting, any disease that have to do with intake and out put.
   In the morning before breakfast

517

3. Which children should have nonoral temperatures taken?

   Oral surgery
   Seizure disorder
   cancer of the mouth
   under six years old
   Child unable to control muscle of mouth to keep it closed.

517

4. Fever, or abnormally high body temperature, is now more often defined as:
   a. An oral temperature of over:

   _100_ ° F or _37.8_ ° C
   b. A rectal temperature of over:

   _100.4_ ° F or _38_ ° C

518

5. When should a child's temperature *not* be taken rectally?

   diarrhea, cancer of rectum, h
   rectopathy
   Under 6 years old

518

6. Why are infants' apical rather than radial pulse rates taken? _To difficult_
   to secure and palpate an accurate radial pulse

518

7. Where should you place the stethoscope when taking an apical pulse rate? How long should you count?

   Left nipple at the sternum
   usually for 30 seconds

518

8. Complete the following chart.

◆◆◆ APPROXIMATE PULSE AND RESPIRATION RATES		
Age	Pulse	Respiration
Birth	30 - 50	110 - 150
4 weeks	26 - 36	100 - 140
4 years	20 - 30	90 - 110
7 years	18 - 26	80 - 100
12 years	16 - 24	76 - 90

518

9. What is the correct-sized cuff to use when taking a child's blood pressure?

2/3 of the arm starting at the shoulder 20 % wider

519

10. List three observations appropriate to each problem area listed below that the nurse can make during the admission procedure.

Problem area	Observation
Growth and Development	
Skin Manifestations	
Neurological System Manifestations	
Other Important Signs and Symptoms	

521   11. List five factors to consider regarding the discharge of a patient.

     a. _Arrangement for transportation_

     b. _dismissal in AM_

     c. _Preplanning & needed teaching_

     d. _Follow up appointments_

     e. _Write specific instructions regarding medications_

516   12. The pediatric nurse should be all of the following *EXCEPT*:
- a. Friendly toward children
- b. A substitute mother
- c. Comfortable with children
- d. A caring professional

516   13. Parents may aid their child during the hospital admission procedure by doing all of the following *EXCEPT*:
- a. Undressing the child
- b. Positioning during temperature taking
- c. Collecting a urine specimen
- d. Checking the child's pulse rate

516   14. The amount of parental participation in the care of the hospitalized child depends on the:
- a. Age of the child
- b. Child's health status
- c. Number of patients assigned to the nurse
- d. Physician's orders

517   15. Parents should be discouraged from bringing the child's personal clothing to the hospital because:
- a. It may have germs
- b. It may not fit
- c. Other children would be jealous
- d. It may get lost

517   16. When speaking to a child, the nurse should:
- a. Crouch down to his eye level
- b. Put her hand on the child's head
- c. Speak loudly and clearly
- d. Talk like the child talks

518   17. The normal pulse range for an infant 2 months old is:
- a. 110 to 150 beats/min
- b. 100 to 140 beats/min
- c. 90 to 120 beats/min
- d. 90 to 110 beats/min

518   18. BP charts can be used to evaluate BP readings obtained and serve over a period of time to demonstrate:
- a. BP variations
- b. Developmental changes
- c. Cultural considerations
- d. Appropriateness for size

518   19. BP measurements in children should be obtained and plotted at least:
- a. Every 6 months
- b. Once every year
- c. Before entering school
- d. Three times per year

520   20. The collection of urine specimens usually is *not* difficult in children who are:
- a. Less than 1 year
- b. Infants
- c. Over 2 1/2 years
- d. Toddlers

520   21. The diet of a newly admitted child is least likely to depend on:
- a. Diagnosis
- b. Age
- c. Allergies
- d. Race

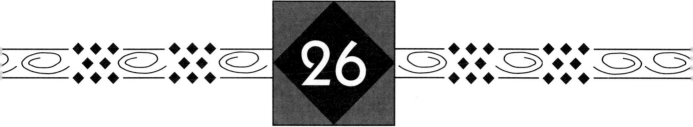

Health Maintenance of the Hospitalized Child

Page Reference

528

1. Before a meal tray is served to a child it should be checked carefully. Name three kinds of observations that should be made.

   a. Any allergies
   b. Developmentally appropriate
   c. Cultral preferences

529

2. Indicate three types of pediatric patients who require very close observation in regard to food intake.

   a. Allergic children
   b. Failure to thrive
   c. Diabetes or metabolic problems

530

3. Jill is 2 years old. Her temperature is 101° F. She cries and turns her head when you ask her to take fluids. What kinds of information would be helpful to you in getting Jill to take on fluids?

   1) What kind of fluids she drinks at home
   2) Can her mother come and feed her
   3) Does she drink from a special cup

191

532

4. The acid-base balance of the blood is maintained in an extremely narrow pH range.

What is the normal pH range? _7.35 - 7.45_

532

5. Which three organs or systems are usually involved in maintaining the acid-base balance of the blood?

a. _Kidney_

b. _Lungs_

c. _Buffer system_

532

6. List four possible clinical manifestations of metabolic acidosis. _- diabetes_

a. _Deep rapid breathing._

b. _Coma_

c. _Weakness_

d. _Apathy, Disorientation_

532

7. Name four conditions that are considered predisposing factors in metabolic acidosis.

a. _Starvation_

b. _Diabetes Mellitus_

c. _Kidney insufficiency_

d. _Severe diarrhea_

533

8. The cardinal principle of fluid balance is _fluid intake must equal fluid output_

534

9. In severe diarrhea, dehydration causes the skin to lose its turgor and to become wrinkled. Why does this happen?

To maintain plasma volume, interstitial fluid shift into the plasm causing wrinkled skin and poor tu

535

10. In infants, severe dehydration associated with 10% body weight loss may be accompanied by what four other signs or symptoms?

a. _Grayish skin_

b. _Rapid & weak pulse_

c. _elevated temp over_

d. _Low Blood pressure_

534

11. Why is the infant more vulnerable to fluid deficit than the adult? Give five reasons.

a. _Poor kidney control_

b. _Takes in and excrete more volume_

c. _High metabolic rate_

d. _T_

e. _____

534

12. List four usual ways that water leaves the body.

a. _Skin_

b. _Lungs_

c. _Kidney_

d. _Intestines_

531-532

13. Match the *electrolyte imbalance* with the *predisposing factor* and the clinical manifestations of imbalance.

Electrolyte imbalance

_d_ K$^+$ ↑ (hyperkalemia)

___ pH ↑ (metabolic alkalosis)

_b_ K$^+$ ↓ (hypokalemia)

_f_ Na$^+$ ↑ (hypernatremia)

_c_ CA^{++} ↓ (hypocalcemia)

_a_ Na$^+$ ↓ (hyponatremia)

**Predisposing factor →
clinical manifestations of imbalance**

a. *Excessive sweating and water inake* → muscular weakness, abdominal cramps, weak rapid pulse

b. *Diarrhea* → hypotension, muscular weakness, weak pulse

c. *Malabsorption syndrome* → tingling, muscular cramping (tetany)

d. *Severe dehydration* → nausea, confusion, muscular weakness

e. *Vomiting (pyloric stenosis)* → depressed, shallow respirations

f. *Dehydration* → dry skin, loss of skin turgor, weight loss, scanty urine

541

14. Play is an important learning activity for every child. Explain four different ways that play can help the child.

a. _Physically_

b. _Emotional_

c. _Intellectually_

d. _Socially_

541   15. The nurse should be able to help the child choose the right kind of play material. List three characteristics that should be kept in mind when choosing toys for any child.

a. _Saftey._

b. _Developmental age_

c. _Durability_

541   16. Why is play so important for the child in the hospital?

Play is a learning activity and is vital to growth

542   17. Complete the play-and-get-well chart on p. 195 by indicating general categories of toys (interest column) and examples of appropriate toys and books that are available on the unit where you are gaining your clinical experience.

543   18. Eighteen-month-old Gena will not take her medicine (5 ml ampicillin). Her mother suggests that you put it in her bottle of milk. How would you respond to this suggestion?

543   19. What other methods of giving the medicine might be suggested to Gena's mother?

Age	Interest	Toys	Books
Infant			
Toddler			
Preschool			
Early school age			
Preadolescent			

543   20. What methods of administration would you consider when giving a 3-month-old infant 2.5 ml phenobarbital? *Syringe, nipple, or rubber-tip medicine dropper.*

545   21. What size needle would you use to give an intramuscular injection to Linda, a 25-lb, 22-month-old toddler? *22 gauge - 1 inch*

544   22. What areas could be used for the injection site? *Vastus lateralis, rectus femoris or deltoid*

544   23. Why would you not consider the gluteal muscle? *because its not well develop and the possibility of damaging the sciatic nerve*

545   24. To facilitate feeding formula to 5-month-old Jackie, normal saline nose drops are ordered 20 minutes before feeding time. His nose is very congested, and his breathing is noisy. How would you clear Jackie's nose of the mucus? *using a bulb syringe, gentle suction*

545   25. How would you administer the nose drops? *The child should be laying c̄ head tilt back over a small pillow or rolled blanket. Medication should be instilled pointed slightly towards the top of the nasal cavity. The child should stay in this position for several minutes*

Maintaining an adequate fluid intake is an important responsibility of the bedside nurse. Three-year-old Paul is recovering from an acute attack of asthma. Paul is begging the doctor to take his intravenous tubing out. The doctor turns to you and says that you can remove it, but adds, "I'm going to count on you to keep Paul well hydrated or the IV will have to be replaced."

---

530   26. What can you do to promote Paul's fluid intake?
Find out what he likes to drink. If possible sit him down while he drinks and offer him a choice

530   27. What fluids should you offer Paul? _depends on Paul allergies_
Popsicles, flavoured ice cubes. Ice cubes
broth, soup, jello, water, milk, -

> Eleven-month-old Ann is receiving an intravenous infusion of 250 ml of 5% dextrose and 0.25 normal saline solution. The infusion has a microdrip chamber, and she is to get 30 ml each hour.

535   28. How fast should the drop rate be? _30 gtts/min_

535-536   29. What are the nurse's responsibilities in relation to Ann's intravenous therapy? Give four considerations.

$\frac{30 \times 60}{1} = \frac{60}{60}$

a. _Child must be appropriatley restraint_
b. _May sure the medicine infusing at the right rate_
c. _Child's response to the fluid therapy_
d. _Check IV site_

> Little John weighed 7 lb 9 oz at birth and is currently 11 months old and weighs 9 lb. He has been on the pediatric unit for 2 weeks. His admission diagnosis was failure to thrive and diarrhea related to his malabsorption syndrome. Recently he has been vomiting after each feeding. He is receiving an intravenous infusion of 5% dextrose in $\frac{1}{3}$ normal saline solution plus electrolytes. He has lost 2 lb since admission. Total parenteral nutrition will be started tomorrow, the day that you will be assigned to his care.

537   30. How does total parenteral nutrition (TPN) differ from conventional pediatric intravenous therapy?

Conventional pediatric intravenous therapy cannot sustain life but TPN can. It has glucose, lipids, fat, minerals and the necessary essential vitamins to promote growth

537   31. Why has the doctor suggested the jugular vein for this particular procedure?

Because the large vein has less risk of thrombosis or phelbities, also dilute the fluids more rapidly

537   32. Can a peripheral vein be used for intravenous alimentation? Is there any danger in the use of such veins?

yes, The danage of tissue damage is greater than when using the jajular vein

537   33. List six essential substances that are provided in TPN.

a. *glucose*

b. *lipids*

c. *vitamins*

d. *protien*

e. *water*

f. *minerals*

524   34. It is *most* important that the child's environment during hospitalization be constantly evaluated to:
a. Maintain order
b. Provide rest
c. Prevent injuries
d. Promote comfort

524   35. Elbow restraints are effective if the child should not:
a. Play
b. Fall
c. Touch his face
d. Reach his feet

528   36. Nuts, raw carrots, and celery should not be served to toddlers because they:
a. Do not like chewy foods
b. Do not have all their teeth
c. May aspirate these foods
d. Should only have liquids

533   37. The amount of fluid that is urged depends on the size and condition of the child. An infant usually takes:
a. 4 bottles/day
b. 100 ml/kg/day
c. 1 quart/day
d. 1500 ml/day

530   38. Infants with active diarrhea and vomiting are usually allowed:
a. Clear fluids
b. Full liquids
c. Nothing by mouth
d. Water

534   39. The largest fluid compartment in the body of a child or adult is the:
              a. Vascular
              b. Interstitial
              c. Extracellular
              d. Intracellular

534   40. Interstitial fluid is similar to plasma except that it contains very little:
              a. Protein
              b. Glucose
              c. Sodium
              d. Potassium

530   41. Positively charged electrolytes are called:
              a. Anions
              b. Buffers
              c. Cations
              d. Molecules

532   42. The acid-base balance of the blood is maintained in an extremely narrow pH range.
              Normally it is:
              a. 7.0 to 7.2
              b. 7.25 to 7.30
              c. 7.35 to 7.45
              d. 7.4 to 7.5

532   43. Blood is normally:
              a. Slightly alkaline
              b. Strongly alkaline
              c. Slightly acid
              d. Strongly acid

532   44. The acid-base balance is normally maintained by all of the following *EXCEPT*:
              a. Lungs
              b. Kidneys
              c. Skin
              d. Buffer systems

533   45. The first fluid storage supply to be tapped as a result of gastrointestinal distur-
              bances is the:
              a. Interstitial fluid
              b. Intracellular fluid
              c. Cerebrospinal fluid
              d. Vascular fluid

534   46. *Moderate* dehydration is characterized by all of the following *EXCEPT*:
              a. Depressed fontanels
              b. Sunken eyeballs
              c. Loss of skin turgor
              d. A weight loss of 10% or higher

543   47. Most medications for children are prepared in liquid form because:
              a. Solutions are easiest to administer
              b. Children are always willing to take a drink
              c. Medicines taste better in liquid
              d. The dose is more accurate

543   48. Before giving any type of ordered medicine, the nurse should always:
       a. Check with the pharmacist
       b. Check with the physician
       c. Check the child's identification
       d. Check the child's age

543   49. The child who takes medicine well always should be:
       a. Rewarded with a toy
       b. Allowed to ambulate
       c. Allowed to play
       d. Praised

545   50. When giving a child a suppository, the nurse should push the medication about:
       a. $1/2$ inch beyond the rectal sphincter
       b. 1 inch beyond the rectal sphincter
       c. $1^1/2$ inches beyond the rectal sphincter
       d. 2 inches beyond the rectal sphincter

545   51. When giving ear drops to a child of 2 years, gently pull the lobe:
       a. Down and back
       b. Up and back
       c. Down and forward
       d. Up and forward

548   52. Nursing notes serve as a permanent record of the patient's treatments, medications, and:
       a. Health status
       b. Cause of illness
       c. Medical progress
       d. Laboratory findings

548   53. The *principles* of charting remain the same in the various hospitals. Good charting for most nurses is:
       a. Automatic
       b. Not difficult
       c. Easy
       d. Learned

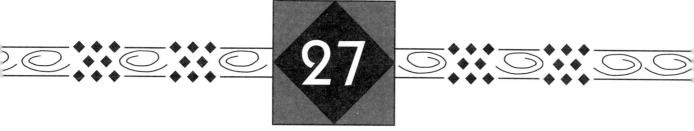

The Child
Experiencing Surgery

Page Reference

551

1. In preparation for your pediatric surgical nursing experience it is important to note certain child-adult distinctions. Discuss the importance of the differences from adults in:

a. Metabolic rate in infants and young children

b. Physical resources in children

c. Healing ability of children

d. Time factor for young children

554   2. a. Indicate four behaviors of an infant or toddler that may demonstrate that he or she is experiencing pain.

(1) _____

(2) _____

(3) _____

(4) _____

556   b. List six different methods (excluding the use of medication) that a parent, nurse, or patient may use to ease pain.

(1) _____

(2) _____

(3) _____

(4) _____

(5) _____

(6) _____

564   3. Nasogastric tubes are used fairly frequently in a surgical area.

a. List two reasons nasogastric suction is used after an operation.

(1) _____

(2) _____

b. Why are nasogastric tubes irrigated? What determines the amount of fluid used?

c. What type of suction is usually ordered for children? _____

_____

562   4. List three methods one can use to determine the position of a gavage tube before beginning a feeding.

a. _____

b. _____

c. _____

560   5. When changing a dressing over a wound, the nurse tries to protect the patient from infection and protect himself or herself from inadvertent contamination. How are these aims fostered? (List three factors.)

a. _____

b. _____

c. _____

551   6. The metabolic rate of infants and young children in comparison to adults is:
        a. Slightly greater
        b. Much greater
        c. Slightly less
        d. Much less

552   7. Food, fluids, and oral medications are withheld before surgery:
        a. For 4 hours
        b. For 6 hours
        c. As ordered
        d. For one night

552   8. Children being admitted for surgery should be especially evaluated for the presence of:
        a. Worms
        b. Birthmarks
        c. Orthopedic anomalies
        d. Respiratory tract infections

554   9. Although infants and toddlers are too young to reveal much about their perception of pain, missing data may be offered by the:
        a. Physician
        b. Parent
        c. Nurse
        d. Sibling

553   10. A child's reaction to pain may be influenced by age, sex, culture, previous experiences, temperament, and the presence of various forms of support. The toddler may respond in several ways but typically the reaction does *not* include:
        a. Aggressive behavior
        b. Descriptive behavior
        c. Regressive behavior
        d. Ritualistic behavior

553   11. When the child returns to the pediatric unit from the recovery room after abdominal surgery, the nurse should check:
        a. Pulse, respiration, and BP
        b. Pulse rate and BP
        c. Pupils and pulse rate
        d. Pupils, pulse rate, and BP

553   12. Following surgery, children should be protected from harming themselves or pulling out needles or tubes by:
        a. Sedation
        b. Constant surveillance
        c. Appropriate restraints
        d. Appropriate positioning

553   13. Judicious ambulation of the postoperative patient aids in the restoration of gastrointestinal functions and helps to prevent:
        a. Pneumonia
        b. Dehydration
        c. Shock
        d. Discomfort

553   14. To aid the child's lung expansion following abdominal surgery, the physician might order:
        a. Cool mist
        b. Chest vibration and clapping
        c. Postural drainage
        d. An incentive spirometer

512   15. Before any intrusive procedure the nurse should prepare the young child, according to the level of understanding:
        a. The day before the procedure
        b. Just before the procedure
        c. During the procedure
        d. The night before the procedure

554   16. Four-year-old Jose is crying because his newly casted arm is hurting. Which of the following pain assessment tools is most desirable to elicit his perception of pain?
        a. Hurt thermometer
        b. Oucher Scale
        c. Visual analog scale
        d. Body diagrams

554   17. When assessing a young child's pain, the nurse must be aware of other factors. Which of the following is least likely to influence what the child is experiencing?
        a. Age
        b. Culture
        c. Doctor
        d. Fear

554   18. The best means of relieving severe pain in children is:
        a. Parenteral narcotics
        b. Antiinflammatory drugs
        c. Muscle relaxants
        d. Oral analgesics

STUDENT'S NAME _____

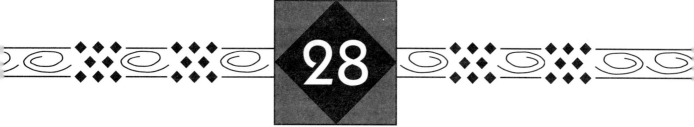

Maintaining Oxygenation

Page Reference

568

1. Label the parts indicated on Fig 28-1.

a. _____   f. _____

b. _____   g. _____

c. _____   h. _____

d. _____   i. _____

e. _____   j. _____

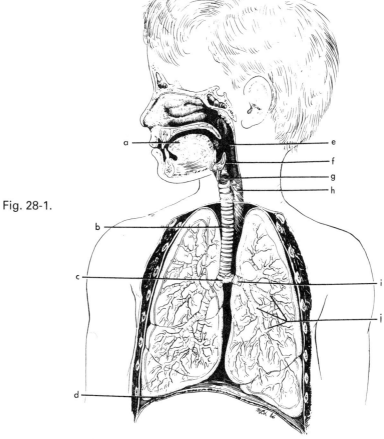

Fig. 28-1.

205

567

2. How does a breakdown in the anatomy or physiology of the respiratory system affect tissues of other organs and systems?

569

3. An infant or child with a respiratory problem in which fluid tends to collect in the chest or abdomen should be placed in what position?

Semi flower position or supported in a car seat.

569

4. What happens to a child's body when more than one third of the hemoglobin is not oxygen saturated?

The child becomes cyanotic

567

5. Any condition that causes a depletion in the ability of the lung tissue to receive air and transfer oxygen and carbon dioxide can cause respiratory distress. List four such conditions.

a. respiratory distress syndrome

b. aspiration

c. Asthma

d. Croup

569

6. List three neurological symptoms that are manifested when a child becomes hypoxic.

a. headache

anxiety

agitation

569-570

7. What is the most accurate way to determine the extent of oxygenation of a patient's blood?

Analyize oxygen and carbon dioxide level in arterial blood sample.

580

8. Explain how the Heimlich maneuver aids in clearing the airway of a patient who is choking.

cause the diaphram to suddenly force air out through the airway

571-572

9. Suction of the naso-oropharyngeal passage and tracheobronchial tree by use of a catheter suction setup is sometimes necessary to clear the airway. List 10 points that should be remembered about this procedure.

a. *Cather size should be equal size if patient*

b. _____

c. _____

d. _____

e. _____

f. _____

g. _____

h. _____

i. _____

j. _____

572

10. What is the best route for long-term airway maintenance when the child needs ventilatory support? *tracheostomy.*

574   11. A child who has a tracheostomy usually cannot speak. List four considerations that can help a 5-year-old child to communicate needs.

   a. _using hand bell. or signal lights_

   b. _magic slate_

   c. _pencil and paper._

   d. _how to put his finger over trach. when he wants to talk._

572   12. Why is it necessary to use sterile technique in the care of a new tracheostomy?

   To preven infecton

577   13. What is the oxygen content of air? _21 %_

577   14. What condition of the eyes sometimes develops as the result of excess oxygen?

   retrolental fibroplasia — Blindness

577   15. What is the most accurate way of assessing the actual oxygen need of a premature infant? _Periodic blood gas determinations_

577   16. How often should the oxygen content in an incubator be checked?

   a. _q 2 h_

   List four of the rules of oxygen administration.

   b. _Place visible no somking sign_

   c. _____

   d. _____

   e. _____

577   17. Besides oxygen, what else can the incubator provide for infants?

   ① _Warmth_

   ② _humidity_

   ③ _easy way to observe infant_

579   18. Describe mouth-to-mouth resuscitation of a child.

Pinch the nose and place mouth

_____

_____

_____

_____

_____

_____

580   19. What items should be available in the hospital for resuscitation emergencies?

_____

_____

_____

_____

584   20. Describe how you would use the Ambu resuscitator on a 6-month-old infant.

_____

_____

_____

_____

_____

_____

_____

580, 584   21. What advantage does the use of the Ambu resuscitator have over mouth-to-mouth resuscitation? _less fatiguing & prevent transmission of disease._

584   22. When are patients placed on mechanical ventilators? (List three instances.)

a. _To maintain possitive pressure in airway_

b. _To reduce the work of breathing_

c. _To treat hypotion hypoxemia_

568   23. List eight signs of respiratory distress in the young child.

a. _____

b. _____

c. _____

d. _____

e. _____

f. _____

g. _____

h. _____

570   24. The most accurate way of determining the extent of oxygenation present is by:
a. Examining the airway with a laryngoscope
b. Oxygen and carbon dioxide blood gas determination
c. Carefully assessing the color of nail beds
d. Monitoring the pulse and respirations

578   25. Warm-mist and steam tents have been replaced because of:
a. Wet linen that must be changed often
b. Difficulty in maintaining them
c. The continued serious danger of burns
d. Fever, which is often present

578   26. A small child in a dense water–aerosol environment must be checked frequently for:
a. Cyanosis
b. Damp clothing
c. Dehydration
d. Choking

575   27. Postural drainage and percussion are most effective when performed after:
a. A trial of epinephrine
b. Meals and before bedtime
c. Aerosol therapy
d. Morning care has been given

577   28. Percussion techniques should not be used over the patient's spine, kidney area, and:
a. Ribs
b. Lateral chest walls
c. Sternum
d. Breast

574   29. A 3-year-old child with a tracheostomy cannot:
a. Eat
b. Drink
c. Cough
d. Talk

576   30. Which of the following is *least* likely to be incorporated with breathing exercises and chest physiotherapy?
- a. Suctioning
- b. Percussion
- c. Vibration
- d. Coughing

574   31. Which of the following medications has been most successful in the treatment of croup?
- a. Vaponefrin
- b. Aminophylline
- c. Proventil
- d. Adrenalin

569   32. Tachycardia and tachypnea are common mechanisms triggered to correct:
- a. Hypoxia
- b. Anxiety
- c. Arrhythmia
- d. Eupnea

570   33. A noninvasive method of measuring oxygen saturation is:
- a. Blood pressure
- b. Pulse oximetry
- c. Oxygen analyzer
- d. Incentive spirometer

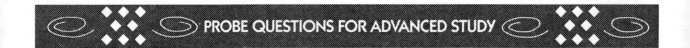

PROBE QUESTIONS FOR ADVANCED STUDY

1. Hospitalization, especially in an intensive care unit, can result in a significant threat to the stability of the family. Knowledge of significant stressors could be used to guide planning and to evaluate the quality of family-centered nursing care. Discuss the Parental Stressor Scale: Pediatric ICU (PSS:PICU) and how it is used to identify parents' most significant stresses. How important are parenting skills during hospitalization? List and briefly describe five coping strategies and/or activities that may reduce parental and child stresses in the PICU setting.

REFERENCES

Heuer L: Parental stressors in a pediatric intensive care unit, *Pediatr Nurs* 19(2):128-133, 1993.

Kramer NA: Comparison of therapeutic touch and casual touch in stress reduction of hospitalized children, *Pediatr Nurs* 16(5):483-485, 1990.

La Montagne LL: Parental coping and activities during pediatric critical care, *Am J Critical Care* 1(2):76-80, 1992.

2. Assessment of pain location, intensity, and quality should become part of the postoperative routine for infants and young children. Infants are neurologically developed enough to perceive pain and to respond to pain. List the most common behaviors manifested by infants in pain. Discuss the physiological indicators of pain in neonates and infants. Why are infants more sensitive to morphine than adults? Discuss the "body outline" as a part of the clinical assessment of pain in children 4 years and older. Do children tell the truth about the pain they are experiencing?

REFERENCES

Eland JM and Coy JA: Assessing pain in the critically ill child, *Focus Crit Care* 17(6):469-475, 1990.

Elander G, Hellstrom G, and Ovarnstrom B: Care of infants after major surgery: observation of behavior and analgesic administration, *Pediatr Nurs* 19(3):221-226, 1993.

Van Cleve LJ and Savedra MC: Pain location: validity and reliability of body outline markings by 4 to 7-year-old children who are hospitalized, Pediatr Nurs 19(3):217-229, 1993.

3. Peripheral venous catheters for administration of medications has become commonplace. The procedure for flushing intermittent access catheters has also become routine with the use of either normal saline or dilute heparin flush. How many units of heparin are recommended as a flush for peripheral IVs in pediatric patients? Why is normal saline being considered for the "standard flush" for intermittent access peripheral venous catheters? What is the most common complication of peripheral venous catheters?

REFERENCES

Cushing M: Hazards of the infiltrated IV, *Am J Nurs* 90(9):31-32, 1990.

Clinical News: Maintaining monitoring lines: yes heparin helps, *Am J Nurs* 93(2):12, 1993.

Danek GD: Pediatric IV catheters: efficacy of saline flush, *Pediatr Nurs* 18(2):111-113, 1992.

4. Maintaining intravenous access in pediatric patients can be challenging. What factors significantly influence peripheral catheter longevity? What is the criteria for considering use of the Port-A-Cath to maintain intravenous access? How often are heparin flushes necessary to maintain the Port-A-Cath when it is not in use? What is meant by extravasation and what are 3 examples?

REFERENCES

Hammond LJ: The Port-A Cath and Per-Q-Cath, *J Pediatr Health Care* 5(1):31-33, 1991.

Millam DA: How to teach good venipuncture technique, *Am J Nurs* 93(7):38-41, 1993.

Wood LS and Gullo SM: IV vesicants: how to avoid extravasation, *Am J Nurs* 93(4):43-46, 1993.

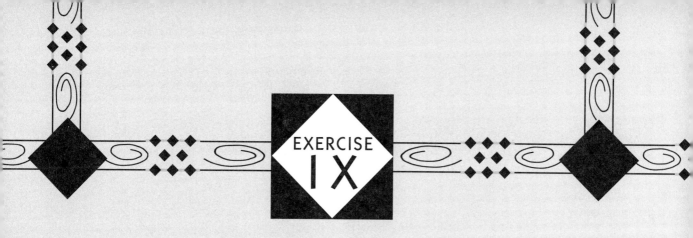

EXERCISE
IX

CHILD HEALTH
PROBLEMS

Although various medical problems and diagnostic tests should not be our focus in nursing, they ake up a significant portion of the pediatric curriculum. Special procedures and tests often must be modiied to conform to the various anatomical, physiological, and psychological differences of children and adolescents. The hospitalization of the child with a ontagious disease presents several medical, social, nd emotional problems, as well as nursing problems. As a student, you will be "exposed" to some of these difficulties. More difficult to treat but usually capable of improvement are those conditions associated with neurological deficit. Chapters 29 through 37 present ome of the most common health problems of children. Knowledge and understanding of these conditions will assist the student in the assessment, planing, and implementation of nursing care.

CLINICAL TIE-IN

What infectious conditions were represented in the clinical area during the past 4 or 5 days? How many were contagious?

2. In the clinical area, what special equipment do you observe that is particularly designed to meet the needs of children with long-term neuromuscular and skeletal problems?

3. An important treatment for children with lung problems is respiratory therapy (RT), given usually after an aerosol treatment. How often do the children on your unit receive RT, and who administers the treatment?

4. What type of code is used in your hospital area to signal the need for immediate medical assistance in cases of cardiac or pulmonary arrest?

5. Who is responsible for teaching self-care to the child with type I insulin-dependent diabetes?

6. Have any patients been admitted recently with a diagnosis of ruptured appendix? How has their postoperative course differed from that of children who underwent an appendectomy without the complication of rupture?

7. Careful examination of a fresh urine specimen is an important diagnostic procedure. How soon are specimens taken to the laboratory for examination?

Alterations in
Body Temperature

Page Reference

589   1. How does the regulation of body temperature through the use of selective therapies help patients? *Brings comfort*

Helps prevent complications that presence in high fever or abnormal fluid loss

590   2. What is the normal range of oral temperature readings? *97.6° – 99°*

590   3. What does normal body temperature in a human represent? *a balance between heat production and heat lost*

591   4. What process is involved in the production of body heat?

Activity of all cells made possible by oxidation or burning of foodstuff within those cells

590
5. How is body heat distributed? _Blood flowing through various parts of the body_

591
6. Cite four ways that body heat can be conserved.

a. _involuntary constriction of the blood vessels of the skin, thus forcing more blood into the warm interior of the body- cutting it off_

from cooler areas of the skin

b. _Automatic reduction of perspiration_

c. _Adding clothing to the body_

d. _Involuntary contraction of the muscle (shivering)_

591
7. What part of the brain is responsible for heat regulation? _hypothalmus_

592
8. Why do children have such wide swings in body temperature?

There temperature regulation is immature or not perfect

meckanism

592
9. What beneficial effects may an elevation in temperature produce?

May help to fight infection and support immune system; warns the individual of the presence of possible disease process

592
10. What often accompanies fever in young children? _Convulsions_

592   11. List four mechanisms by which an infant can lose body heat, and give an example of each.

failure to dry an infant during a bath or immediately after

a. <u>Evaporation</u> —

b. <u>Conduction</u> — *baby contact with cold examining table or scale*

c. <u>Convection</u> — *exposure to draft cool oxygen flow esp in the face*

d. <u>Radiation</u> — *his proximity to cold walls and other objects*

593   12. Why is heat conservation so important in the care of small infants?

To conserve calories, avoiding weight loss and acidosis

593   13. In what situation might *deep* hypothermia be employed intentionally?

For children on going cardiac or thoracic surgery

589   14. A child may be hospitalized for a diagnostic work-up when a fever of unknown origin (FUO) persists for:
a. More than 1 day
b. More than 2 days
c. More than 3 days
d. More than 5 days

589   15. Appropriate temperature maintenance may be particularly critical for small infants by conserving calories and:
a. Increasing feedings
b. Preventing hyperglycemia
c. Increasing oxygenation
d. Preventing acidosis

591   16. The centigrade equivalent of average oral body temperature is:
a. 35.2°   c. 37.0°
b. 36.4°   d. 38.0°

590   17. An accurate and less invasive temperature route especially favored for infants and young children is:
a. Rectal   c. Axillary
b. Skin   d. Oral

591   18. Core temperatures are those measured near:
a. Arteries
b. The heart
c. Veins
d. The head

591   19. Body heat is conserved by the automatic reduction of perspiration by:
a. Involuntary constriction of blood vessels
b. Decreasing metabolism
c. Involuntary dilation of blood vessels
d. Decreasing activity

592   20. A medical term that means feverish or caused by fever is:
         a. Hypothermia
         b. Febrile
         c. Hyperglycemic
         d. Seizure

592   21. A child may have an elevation in temperature during a prolonged episode of:
         a. Coughing
         b. Feeding
         c. Sleeping
         d. Crying

592   22. Excessive heat production by the body not involving an elevation in temperature set-point may be associated with:
         a. Infection
         b. Hyperthyroidism
         c. Allergy
         d. Malignancy

593   23. Cellular metabolism in the absence of adequate oxygen produces:
         a. Alkalosis
         b. Dehydration
         c. Acidosis
         d. Perspiration

594   24. Priority should be given to which one of the following methods of lowering body temperature:
         a. Administration of fluids
         b. Removal of clothing
         c. Administration of antipyretics
         d. Tepid sponge bath

593   25. The temperature inside an incubator necessary to conserve the infant's energy depends on several factors. Which one of the following *is not* a consideration in setting the temperature?
         a. Gestational age
         b. Weight
         c. Physical appearance
         d. Age following birth

594   26. Medications might be ordered to help reduce fever. Such medications are called:
         a. Antibiotics
         b. Antibacterials
         c. Antipyretics
         d. Antihistamines

594   27. Temperature-reducing medications are not ordered for low grade fevers. The nurse knows that a low grade fever is one that is usually considered to be not more than:
         a. 99° F (37.2° C)   c. 101° F (38.3° C)
         b. 100° F (37.8° C)   d. 102° F (38.9° C)

593   28. A tepid water tub or sponge bath may be administered to reduce fever. The recommended beginning temperature of the water in the tub is approximately:
         a. 68° F (20.0° C)   c. 88° F (31.1° C)
         b. 78° F (25.5° C)   d. 98° F (36.6° C)

Skin Problems

age Reference

599

1. How does the skin aid in the regulation of body temperature?

   Principally through capillary dialation & constriction and forming a cooling pespiration

600

2. Match the names of skin conditions with their characteristics.

   _____ A flat spot or stain, such as a freckle

   _____ A small, solid elevation on the skin, such as a pimple

   _____ A small elevation of the skin obviously containing fluid, such as a blister

   _____ A pus-filled vesicle

   _____ A raw area often depressed or forming a cavity, caused by loss of normal covering tissue

   a. Vesicle
   b. Macule
   c. Pustule
   d. Ulcer
   e. Papule

600

3. List seven points that should be included in the description of a skin lesion.

   a. Size
   b. Elevation
   c. Quality
   d. Color
   e. Distribution
   f. Associated sensory disturbances
   g. Type of drainage or exudate noted

219

602

4. List four situations that often predispose an infant to diaper rash.

a. _poorly washed and rinsed diapers_

b. _infrequent diaper changes_

c. _prolonged use of plastic covers_

d. _incomplete or infrequent washing & drying_

602

5. What measures can be taken to prevent diaper rash?

a. _To use of gentle antiseptic final rinse_

b. _Careful washing & drying of diaper area._

Amber Reed was admitted to the children's unit last evening with atopic dermatitis. She is 5 months old and weighs 17 lb. Her entire body is reddened and covered with small weeping vesicles. In some places crusts or scales are visible. Her face is some-what swollen. Mrs. Reed is at the cribside. The physician's orders include: ProSobee formula ad lib, daily Aveeno bath, and trimmed fingernails. In preparation for your assignment your instructor asks you the following questions.

602

6. What is meant by atopic dermatitis? _most common manifest-ation of allergic disease in infancy_

602

7. How does one so small become exposed to allergens? _By ingestion, inhalation, By contact_

603

8. Is eczema inherited? _There is often a family history of all_

603

9. To successfully treat eczema, what must you do as soon as possible? _Identify the offending allergens_

603

10. List eight common items that can harbor allergens to which Amber might be sensitive.

a. _dust_

b. _toys_

c. _stuff animals_

d. _books_

e. _Plants_

f. _drapes_

g. _rugs_

h. _____

603 11. What is Aveeno, and why was it ordered for Amber's bath?

603 12. Later, when you are caring for Amber, her mother tells you that she has been washing Amber several times a day with soap. She asks if the soap made her baby's skin red. How would you answer this question?

603 13. Mrs. Reed asks you why you are cutting the baby's nails. Explain why it is necessary to cut them.

603 14. When do you think it would be best to cut Amber's fingernails? _____

       _____

454 15. Mrs. Reed asks you about immunizations. She tells you that Amber has not been immunized because of her skin. How would you respond?

607 16. Name two causes of burns in toddlers.

       a. _Hot coffee_____

       b. _Hot tub_____

607   17. Name two causes of burns in older children.

a. _Using kerosene oil_

b. _Clothes caught on fire while playing o match_

607   18. Burns are classified into three categories, depending on the depth of penetration of the body surface. Describe:

a. Superficial burns _Epidermis - Partial thickness._
1st degree, Superficial, tender, slightly
swollen recued

b. Partial-thickness burns _Dermis & Epidermis Partial_
thickness, 2nd degree - Some nerve ending
in tact.

c. Full thickness burns _Dermis, Epidermis portions & subcata_
tissue,   _full thickness   3th degree burn._
Leathery appearance little moisture.

608   19. Describe how you would extinguish the flames on the nightclothes of a 4-year-old boy. _If water ready, available it should be used_
If not wrap him in a blanket, or throw rug
to smother the flames.
If not.   Stop, drop, Roll.

608   20. How would you prepare the child to take him to the hospital?
Burn area should be rinsed   immediatly
with cold water if possible quickly
transport child clean sheet & blanket

Ten-year-old Steve has just arrived in the emergency room with what appear to be full-thickness burns on his chest, arms, and legs.

609   21. What are the two most important principles to remember in the care of this child?

a. _Prevention of shock_

b. _Maintaining an open airway_

608-609   22. When the physician rushes to Steve's bedside, he is carrying a mask, which he quickly puts on. Why did he put a mask on, and what should you do?

> When you return, the physician gives you his written orders and asks that you take them to the charge nurse immediately. He states that he is calling for an ear, nose, and throat and plastic surgery consultation. The physician's orders read:
> NPO
> Blood gases stat
> CBC—cross and type
> #1 IV—600 ml Ringer's lactate at 200 ml first hour
> #14 Foley catheter to gravity drainage
> #14 nasogastric tube
> Vital signs, including BP q 30 min
> I and O q l hr with specific gravity
> Tetanus toxoid, 0.5 ml IM if 5 years has elapsed since last dose
> Weight
> 500,000 units aqueous penicillin q 6 h IV
> Strict isolation
> Demerol 25 mg IV stat

609   23. Why did the physician order that Steve be given nothing by mouth and have a nasogastric tube inserted?

609   24. What specific nursing measure aids in determining the role of intravenous fluid and provides an index of Steve's general condition?

_____

_____

609   25. Infection is a common but very serious complication in any burned patient. What three measures has the physician taken to try to prevent this from happening?

a. Tetanous toxiod

b. Strict Isolation

c. Peninullin

609   26. The Demerol helps to control shock, but why is there more pain accompanying a partial-thickness burn than a full-thickness burn? Because in partial-thickness some of the nerve ending is still intact

> The physician tells you that he will wash Steve's burns in the operating room. After primary excision he plans to apply porcine heterografts.

610   27. What does the physician mean by primary excision?

610   28. What are the advantages of porcine heterografts for Steve?

Use to cover the wound and prevent infection in the preparation for autografts

600   29. Which one of the following is not considered part of the integumentary system?
a. Hair   c. Nails
b. Mucous glands   d. Sweat glands

600   30. The skin functions in many ways to protect the individual. However, it has limited powers of:
a. Sensation of heat   c. Sensation of coldness
b. Fluid loss   d. Fluid absorption

600   31. A small elevation of the skin obviously containing fluid, such as a blister, is known as a:
a. Crust   c. Vesicle
b. Papule   d. Pustule

600   32. A moist circumscribed skin lesion that often is depressed is called:
            a. Abrasion   c. Ulcer
            b. Erosion   d. Crust

600   33. A common pediatric problem caused by a blockage of the sweat pores is known as:
            a. Intertrigo   c. Eczema
            b. Seborrheic dermatitis   d. Miliaria rubra

601   34. A condition that is characterized by a scaly eruption on an inflammatory base and
            that chiefly affects the scalp, eyebrows, eyelids, and pubic region is:
            a. Seborrheic dermatitis   c. Chafing
            b. Eczema   d. Scabies

602   35. Infants with diaper rash are felt to have an irritant dermatitis, but another consid-
            eration is:
            a. Eczema   c. Seborrhea
            b. Intertrigo   d. Impetigo

604   36. Which one of the following skin conditions is caused by a beta-hemolytic strepto-
            coccus organism and is characterized by small blisters that become filled with pus
            and eventually break, causing thick yellow-red crusts?
            a. Impetigo   c. Herpes simplex
            b. Eczema   d. Acne

604   37. Which one of the following is caused by a fungus that attacks the hair base, causing
            it to break and leaving areas of baldness?
            a. Eczema   c. Scabies
            b. Tinea capitis   d. Tinea versicolor

605   38. Which of the following types of ringworm is essentially limited to the postpubes-
            cent child?
            a. Tinea pedis   c. Tinea capitis
            b. Tinea cruris   d. Tinea corporis

605   39. Pediculosis capitis is an infestation of the hair of the head by lice. A medication
            that is highly effective in the treatment of this condition is:
            a. Desenex   c. Kwell
            b. Povan   d. Acyclovir

606   40. Acne vulgaris is a common skin inflammation among boys and girls. When acne is
            present, it first appears almost without exception during:
            a. Prepuberty   c. Adolescence
            b. Puberty   d. Late adolescence

609   41. The shock phase of the body's response to extensive burns usually is considered to
            last from:
            a. 24 to 48 hours   c. 48 to 72 hours
            b. 36 to 60 hours   d. 60 to 72 hours

609   42. Which one of the following actions should be taken *first* when moderate or major
            burns are present?
            a. Fluid replacement   c. Control of bleeding
            b. Maintenance of an airway   d. Administration of pain medication

610   43. Which one of the following procedures is necessary to relieve compression from a circumferential burn that has formed a thick black crust?
a. Debridement
b. Escharotomy
c. Excision
d. Grafting

610   44. When devitalized burned tissue is cut away down to the fascia, the procedure is called:
a. Primary excision
b. Devitalization
c. Escharotomy
d. Debridement

610   45. Grafts from another part of the patient's own body are known as:
a. Heterografts
b. Autografts
c. Homografts
d. Biological dressings

612   46. Mortality caused by infection has declined as a result of the effectiveness of improved topical antibacterial agents. Which one of the following topical agents is painless on application?
a. Sulfamylon
b. Betadine
c. Silver sulfadiazine
d. Silver nitrate

612   47. A topical medication that has greatly reduced the incidence of infection but can cause metabolic acidosis is:
a. Betadine
b. Silver nitrate
c. Sulfamylon acetate
d. Silver sulfadiazine

614   48. Burned extremities should never be allowed to assume long periods of:
a. Flexion
b. Extension
c. Abduction
d. Rotation

614   49. If children consider themselves responsible for their own injuries, they might be preoccupied with feelings of:
a. Anxiety
b. Fear
c. Guilt
d. Helplessness

612   50. To provide for growth and tissue repair, the child with large burns probably will be maintained on a regimen of:
a. Intravenous glucose
b. Whole blood and plasma
c. Tube feedings
d. Plasma expanders

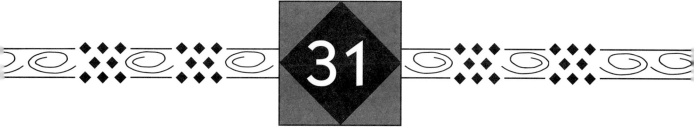

Infectious Disorders

Page Reference

619-620

1. Match the terms in the righthand column with the definitions in the lefthand column.

_____ Formation of protective antibodies as
the result of having the disease
_____ Disorder that can be passed directly
from person to person
_____ The way that organisms gain entrance
into a person's body
_____ Time of exposure until the appearance
of signs or symptoms of the disease
_____ Observance of certain barrier techniques
designed to stop the spread of illness
_____ An infection acquired during
hospitalization
_____ Immediate protection of a short duration
against a certain disease
_____ Preparation that, when introduced into the
body, causes the formation of antibodies
against a certain type of organism

a. Vaccine
b. Passive immunity
c. Portal of entry
d. Isolation
e. Incubation period
f. Contagious disease
g. Nosocomial infection
h. Active immunity

617

2. Why is the use of infection precautions in the hospital necessary?

a. _For the saftey of patients, visitors and staff_

b. _____

617

3. What is the rationale for the use of certain barrier techniques in the hospital?

Based on knowledge of how contagious disease is transmitted — the chain of infection

618   4. Describe five role functions of the (ICP) in the hospital.

a. Keep records and rate of infect

b. Helps interpret & prepare protocols for many hospital practices including isolation precau

c. Conducts examinations of appropriate interventions to reduce risks

d. Proposes investigations to determine reasons for difficulty in patient care practices associated c̄ skin infection

e. Consultant and educational resource.

619   5. The study of the occurrence, distribution, and causes of health and disease in humans is known as ___epidemology___.

619   6. During which phase of a disease is the patient usually most infectious?

Second phase called prodrome

620   7. A place where microorganisms live and multiply is called ___reservior of infecti___

619   8. Which infectious patient is potentially the most dangerous to the caregivers and other patients?

The person who is in the second phase of the prodrome phase.

623   9. List four desirable characteristics of the caregiver related to the transmission of contagious disease in the hospital.

a. Free from communicable infections

b. Knowledge regarding possible special need to reevaluate assignment.

c. Cognizant of the need to maintain good general health.

d. Knowledge and dependable regarding infections precautions needed -

623

10. List four general health habits that help to prevent disease.

    a. Proper nutrition

    b. Adequate rest

    c. Good personal hygiene

    d. Use of stress reduction techniques.

623

11. The most important procedure in preventing the spread of infection is hand washing. Describe the technique of hand washing.

    Handwashing - a vigorous, systemic, brief rubbing together of all surfaces of lathered hands, followed by rinsing under a stream of water.

624-625

12. In addition to the furniture needed in all standard patient units, a unit where an infectious patient is cared for should include the following seven items:

    a. Sink c running water & toilet

    b. Box of gloves

    c. Mask & gowns, eye protection

    d. Hand washing agent · antimicrobial.

    e. Paper towels

    f. Laundry hamper

    g. Plastic bag for collection of trash.

625

13. What factors influence who can visit an infectious patient?

    Type of isolation order - patient & visitor in consideration

619

14. List four different ways that infectious diseases may be transmitted.

    a. Vector borne - insect

    b. man - common

    c. Direct or Indirect droplet

    d. Airborne

15. Complete the chart below.

Disease	Infectious agent	Mode of transmission	Communicable period	Incubation period	Prevention
Bacillary dysentery					
Chickenpox					
Rubella					
Measles					

628

640

628

632

Meningococcal meningitis				
Infectious mononucleous				
Mumps				
Hepatitis (HAV)				

632 Meningococcal meningitis

634 Infectious mononucleous

634 Mumps

630 Hepatitis (HAV)

620

16. Many of the government recommendations involving isolation techniques and methods of disease control now originate in the:
    a. Children's Bureau, Washington, D.C.
    b. Centers for Disease Control and Prevention, Atlanta, Ga.
    c. National Institutes of Health, Bethesda, Md.
    d. Department of Public Health, Washington, D.C.

619-620

17. An example of a disease that is infectious but not contagious is:
    a. Rabies
    b. Pyelonephritis
    c. Congenital rubella syndrome
    d. Hepatitis (HAV)

620

18. Which one of the following is associated with nosocomial infections?
    a. Administration of medicines
    b. Family visitation
    c. Colostomy care
    d. Urinary catheterization

623

19. The *one* isolation precaution that always is employed when caring for an infected patient is:
    a. Isolation gowns
    b. Gloves
    c. Hand washing
    d. Masks

453

20. The protection that young infants have against certain diseases is obtained from the mother and lasts for about:
    a. 1-3 months
    b. 2-4 months
    c. 3-5 months
    d. 4-6 months

628

21. Which pair indicated below is incorrect?
    a. Shigellosis—bacillary dysentery
    b. German measles—rubeola
    c. Chickenpox—varicella
    d. Typhoid fever—enteric fever

453

22. Protective substances that can form in the body as a result of contact with infectious or foreign agents are known as:
    a. Antigens
    b. Allergens
    c. Antibodies
    d. Vaccines

456

23. Current practice begins DPT immunization when the infant is:
    a. 1 month of age
    b. 2 months of age
    c. 3 months of age
    d. 4 months of age

457
24. After the initial series of immunizations, *booster doses* are given to:
a. Maintain maximum immunity
b. Protect against new strains of infection
c. Destroy the disease-producing agent
d. Establish new antibodies against disease

454
25. A two-dose measles schedule is recommended for children, and the first dose for those in high-risk areas should be given at:
a. 6 months of age
b. 12 months of age
c. 15 months of age
d. 18 months of age

454
26. The second measles vaccine is routinely recommended between ages:
a. 12-15 months
b. 15-18 months
c. 18-24 months
d. 4-6 years

458
27. Pertussis immunization should not be repeated if there is a history of fever greater than 105° F (40.5° C) and if which one of the following has been reported:
a. Weight loss
b. Seizures
c. Diaper rash
d. Eczema

458
28. There has been much controversy about immunizing children of pregnant women, but children should be given rubella vaccine because:
a. The risk of the disease is greater in infants
b. There is no passive immunity against rubella
c. The vaccine virus is not communicable
d. The disease may be more significant to adults

628
29. A rose-colored macular rash occurring first on the face, then on the other body parts, and associated with enlarged, tender lymph nodes indicates:
a. Scarlet fever
b. Measles
c. Rubella
d. Chickenpox

632-633
30. A spinal tap and culture is needed to confirm the diagnosis of:
a. Infectious mononucleosis
b. Staphylococcal infection
c. Meningitis
d. Varicella zoster

641
31. Vaccines are routinely recommended for all of the following diseases *EXCEPT*:
a. Measles
b. Chickenpox
c. Polio
d. Mumps

635

32. Lifelong immunity usually follows the first attack of:
    a. Streptococcal infections
    b. Mumps
    c. Gonorrhea
    d. Staphylococcal infections

621, 640

33. Children with which one of the following contagious problems would be placed on "transmission-based precautions" in the hospital?
    a. Congenital rubella syndrome
    b. Impetigo
    c. Pertussis
    d. Hepatitis (HAV and HBV)

621, 640

34. Children with which one of the following contagious problems would be placed on "transmission-based precautions" in the hospital setting?
    a. Infectious parotitis
    b. Tetanus
    c. Pulmonary tuberculosis
    d. Varicella

640

35. The virus causing chickenpox can also cause:
    a. Zoster
    b. Impetigo
    c. Herpes simplex
    d. Variola

Neurosensory and Musculoskeletal Disorders

Page Reference

652

1. Make the best match of the following orthopedic terms and definitions.

_____ a _____ Epiphyseal arrest

_____ c _____ Rotational osteotomy

_____ b _____ Arthroplasty

_____ d _____ Arthrodesis

a. Bone stapling
b. Joint reconstruction
c. Realignment
d. Joint stabilizer

665

2. List two medications commonly used by children who have seizures.

a. Dilantin , Phenobarbital

b. Tegertool

668

3. The child with cerebral palsy might have a very minor muscular problem, or the child might have such severe motor neuron damage that he or she is completely dependent on others for all needs. List five possible causes of cerebral palsy.

a. Pressure on brain

b. Cerebral anoxia

c. Direct injury

d. Embolus

e. Hemmorhage

Infection of brain
Toxcity of brain

658   4. Spinal curvatures can result from several types of stress and can develop in various directions. The three major types of abnormal spinal curves and their definitions are:

a. _Scolosis = S-shaped lateral curvature_

b. _Lordosis — exageerated lumbar_

c. _Kyphosis — humpback_

658   5. Four conditions that can cause paralytic scoliosis are:

a. _Poliomylitis_

b. _Myelingocele_

c. _Duchenne - muscular dystrophy_
   Other nueromuscular disorder

660-661   6. Youngsters who have more serious and progressive curvatures usually are candidates for spinal fusion. What kinds of nursing observations are necessary in the care of a patient with a new spinal fusion? (List four considerations.)

a. _Observation of voiding, stool, dressing_

b. _Respiratory systems_

c. _Nuerologic symptoms_

661   7. Discuss the nursing care that is especially appropriate for a child who has had a spinal fusion.

a. _Careful positioning log rolling_

b. _Nuerologic observation_

c. _Fluids decreased_

d. _Turn cough & deep breathe_

660   8. What is a Harrington rod, and where might it be placed?

An internal rod place in the spinal column for spinal correction

660   9. What is the role of the Milwaukee brace in the management of scoliosis?

To Use as an nonoperative measures to correct spinal curvatures.

660   10. Complete union and maturation at a spinal fusion site may take about ____/_____

_____year_____

> It was a balmy spring day and happy Colleen went to the backyard to swing. Fifteen minutes later this blond, pony-tailed 6-year-old was found crying and crumpled in the dirt, her right leg angled strangely beneath her. Colleen had managed to sustain an oblique fracture of the midportion of the large thigh bone. No bony fragment pierced the skin.

649   11. Identify her fracture by placing an X on Fig. 32-1.

649   12. Label the most characteristic fracture of childhood by placing a Y on the shaft of the appropriately fractured bone (bottom of Fig. 32-1).

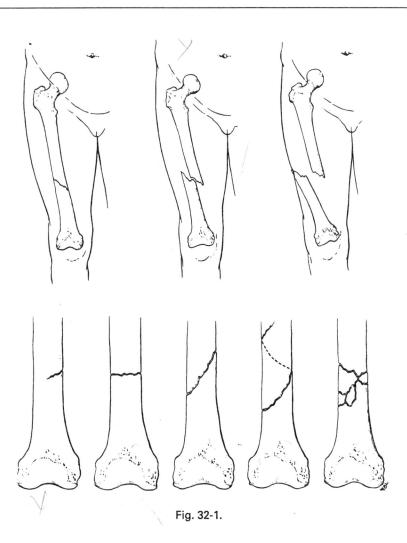

Fig. 32-1.

An ambulance was called, and after Colleen's leg was splinted she got her first ride to the hospital in an ambulance, though she regretted later that no one put on the siren. Dr. Carpenter met Colleen and her parents at the emergency room. He said that Colleen would have to stay at the hospital in a type of balanced traction maintained by a Steinmann pin.

651, 693

13. What does this information tell you about the following?

   a. The fracture itself _needed reduction. An open reduction might performed. More weight probably necessary_

651, 698

   b. Colleen's ability to move in bed _Used the overhead trapeze, sit up in bed; could turn slightly towards broken leg while supine_

694-695

   c. Colleen's orthopedic nursing needs (list six)

   (1) _good position_
   (2) _Skin care_
   (3) _cough & deep breathing_
   (4) _Check for circulation_
   (5) _Check for constipation_
   (6) _Increased fluid intake_

Janine Jacobs is a 17-month-old infant suffering from intermittent generalized tremors of unknown origin, which began 3 months ago and have become increasingly frequent. She has been admitted to the medical center for a more extensive diagnostic workup and treatment evaluation.

663

14. What equipment should be available at the bedside of this child?
   Side rails; padded crib rails

663

15. What should you do if Janine suddenly becomes rigid, with her eyes rolling back in her head?
   Turn her to the side, keep from injury don't restrain her

663

16. What aspects of the seizure should you observe? (List five points.)

   a. _Time it started & what preceeded it_
   b. _Duration_

c. *How it progress* _____

d. *the need for suctioning - oxygen* _____

e. *Position of the eyes* _____

663

17. Would you be able to report if Janine has an aura? *No it's* _____

subjective _____

_____

> Tim Johnson suffered brain damage as a result of high bilirubin filters secondary to Rh incompatibility as an infant. His vision is impaired, and he has a moderate hearing loss. He demonstrates athetoid-type motions as he sits in his chair in the special education classroom of the orthopedic center.

670

18. What kind of movement would be described as athetoid?

anthetoid — r _____

669

19. Tim Johnson's problems are extensive and require a team approach to provide comprehensive care. List 10 members of the professional team that might be required to provide care and guidance for him.

a. _____

b. _____

c. _____

d. _____

e. _____

f. _____

g. _____

h. _____

i. _____

j. _____

Fifteen-year-old Susan Jenson could not get her dresses to fit right anymore. Her hems would never hang straight, and the shoulders did not look as they should. One day her gym instructor, Mrs. Allen, asked to see her privately in her office. Mrs. Allen suggested that Susan see the school nurse. The nurse inspected her spine in the three screening positions. The outcome of the examination let her to contact Susan's parents about an orthopedic evaluation. One week later Susan was fitted for a Milwaukee brace. She was being treated for idiopathic scoliosis.

659

20. According to most references, Susan's spinal curvature must have been at least

    _____ $20°$ _____ degrees.

660

21. When should Susan wear the brace?

    All the time except for time devoted to hygiene

648

22. When a child's bone is fractured and a portion of the bone remains intact, the fracture is called:
    a. Greenstick
    b. Spiral
    c. Oblique
    d. Comminuted

648

23. A nurse encountering a child with unknown injuries who has been in an automobile accident should take which action *first*:
    a. Control bleeding
    b. Send for help
    c. Assess for fractures
    d. Establish an airway

651

24. First-aid treatment for a possible fracture should include:
    a. Stabilizing the part
    b. Keeping the part warm
    c. Elevating the part
    d. Administering pain medication

651

25. When a child's fractured femur is reduced, a certain amount of *overriding* may be necessary to prevent:
    a. Infection
    b. Excessive growth
    c. Swelling
    d. Muscle spasm

697

26. Bryant's traction is useful in treating lower extremity fractures of infants and toddlers weighing:
    a. Less than 30 lb
    b. More than 20 lb
    c. Less than 40 lb
    d. More than 40 lb

Neurosensory and Musculoskeletal

STUDENT'S NAME _____

653   27. Torticollis refers to:
          a. Paralysis of the brachial plexus
          b. Fracture of the wrist
          c. Shortening of the neck muscle
          d. Fracture of the clavicle

662   28. Absence seizures can be:
          a. Characterized by a relatively brief loss of consciousness
          b. Initiated by exposure to darkness
          c. Controlled by hyperventilation
          d. Characteristically predicted by the appearance of an aura

668   29. Residual complications from meningitis can include all of the following *EXCEPT*:
          a. Encephalitis
          b. Hydrocephalus
          c. Learning problem
          d. Mental insufficiency

680   30. Amblyopia refers to:
          a. Loss of visual acuity
          b. Distorted visual image
          c. Hereditary visual problems
          d. Traumatic eye injury

653   31. Which of the following diagnostic procedures or signs is used to identify Duchenne's muscular dystrophy?
          a. Kernig's sign
          b. Creatinine phosphokinase levels   ⊂ PK
          c. Mucous membrane
          d. Sedimentation rate

653   32. The onset of Duchenne's muscular dystrophy usually occurs between:
          a. 1 and 3 years of age
          b. 2 and 4 years of age
          c. 3 and 6 years of age
          d. 4 and 7 years of age

653   33. Duchenne's muscular dystrophy is a hereditary condition that affects males; the pattern of inheritance is:
          a. Autosomal dominant
          b. Sex-linked dominant
          c. Autosomal recessive
          d. Sex-linked recessive

656   34. Juvenile rheumatoid arthritis manifests itself with swollen, stiff, painful joints. Which one of the following is the drug of choice to relieve pain and reduce swelling?
          a. Gold salts
          b. Aspirin
          c. Ibuprofen
          d. Tylenol

656   35. Steroid therapy might be used in rare instances in the treatment of juvenile rheumatoid arthritis. However, prolonged steroid therapy can cause undesirable side effects including all of the following *EXCEPT*:
   - a. Mental retardation
   - b. "Moon face"
   - c. Hirsutism
   - d. Skeletal decalcification

658   36. The diagnosis of osteosarcoma is made only after:
   - a. X-ray studies
   - b. Cultures
   - c. CAT scan
   - d. Biopsy

672   37. Medulloblastomas typically grow rapidly, causing early remarkable signs and symptoms of intracranial pressure, which can include:
   - a. Falling BP
   - b. Rising pulse
   - c. Constricted pupils
   - d. Increased BP

658   38. Idiopathic scoliosis, an S-shaped curvature of the spine:
   - a. Is most common in adolescent boys
   - b. Probably involves genetic factors
   - c. Is best detected by screening in high school
   - d. May cause neurological disease

658   39. The progression of the S-shaped curvature is usually:
   - a. Slow
   - b. Unpredictable
   - c. Painful
   - d. Rapid

657   40. A developmental disease of the hip commonly seen in children between the ages of 4 and 8 years:
   - a. Congenital dislocated hip
   - b. Osteomyelitis
   - c. Legg-Calvé-Perthes disease
   - d. Osteosarcoma

657   41. Osteomyelitis is an inflammation of the bone resulting chiefly from the infectious agent:
   - a. *H. influenzae*
   - b. B hemolytic streptococcus
   - c. *Staphylococcus aureus*
   - d. *Mycobacterium tuberculosis*

674   42. A neuroblastoma is an undifferentiated malignant tumor arising from the adrenal medulla or from:
   - a. Parasympathetic ganglia
   - b. Lymphatic tissue
   - c. Connective tissue
   - d. Sympathetic ganglia

674   43. In addition to neurologic manifestations, children with neuroblastoma often initially have varied constitutional symptoms including all of the following *EXCEPT*:
        a. Weight loss
        b. Hypotension
        c. Anorexia
        d. Anemia

674   44. A favorable prognosis can be expected when a localized neuroblastoma is diagnosed before:
        a. 2 years of age
        b. 6 years of age
        c. 10 years of age
        d. 14 years of age

675   45. About 17% of children admitted to the hospital with head trauma have a fractured skull. What percentage of these children have active intracranial bleeding?
        a. 1%
        b. 10%
        c. 25%
        d. 50%

677   46. About 75% of epidural hematomas are associated with:
        a. Abdominal bleeding
        b. Brain stem injury
        c. Skull fracture
        d. Retrograde amnesia

677   47. A hematoma that is caused by rupture of the low-pressure bridging of veins in the space under the dura is called:
        a. Epidural
        b. Subdural
        c. Subarachnoid
        d. Cerebellar

675   48. Intracranial pressure might begin to rise when brain trauma is associated with:
        a. Fever
        b. Unconsciousness
        c. Bleeding
        d. Amnesia

675   49. Increasing intracranial pressure in the school age child is manifested by a deterioration in the state of consciousness and:
        a. Rising systemic BP
        b. Increased pulse
        c. Falling systemic BP
        d. Increased respirations

675   50. Like other tissues, when the brain is subjected to injury it becomes:
        a. Infected
        b. Necrotic
        c. Edematous
        d. Painful

678

51. Surgical intervention is usually required when the head- injured child has sustained:
    a. Linear skull fracture
    b. Contusion
    c. Depressed skull fracture
    d. Concussion

678

52. Cerebrospinal fluid leaking from the ear or nose causes increased concern because of the danger of:
    a. Hemorrhage
    b. Meningitis
    c. Cerebral anoxia
    d. Hydrocephalus

678

53. Following a head injury, the most frequent cause of death is:
    a. Hypotensive shock
    b. Cerebral anoxia
    c. Cerebral edema
    d. Ruptured spleen

676

54. A neurological check includes all of the following *EXCEPT*:
    a. Vital signs
    b. Level of consciousness
    c. Pupillary signs
    d. Blood gases

679

55. When serial examinations of the head-injured child suggest that intracranial pressure is increasing, fluid intake should be:
    a. Increased
    b. Discontinued
    c. Restricted
    d. Forced

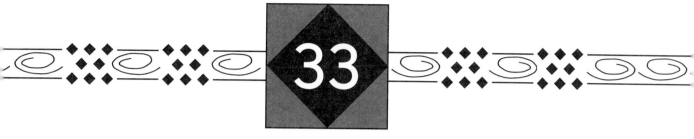

Orthopedic Technology

age Reference

693   1. Often traction or methods of exerting pull must precede casting. List four reasons for traction.

a. Prevent muscle spasm & pain

b. Reduction of fracture — dislocated

c. Stabilize in injured part

d. To prevent deformities

694   2. Describe skin traction.

Skin traction helps position the bone indirectly by pulling the muscle & skin.

It is relatively simple and involves no surgical operation

694   3. What are the two disadvantages of skin traction?

a. Can be irritating to the skin

b. Supportive wrapping may cause allergies

694   4. How is skeletal traction secured?

By inserting mechanical devices such as wire, tongs, pins through the bone and attaching prescribe weight.

245

694

5. What are two main disadvantages of skeletal traction?

a. Since the bone is pierced, danger of infection is present

b. The insertion area for drainge, oder & signs of inflammation.

694

6. How is traction maintained?

Pull in one direction must be balanced by pull in opposite direction (countertraction) for traction to be ~~efficently~~ effectuely maintain

694

7. What are the four basic ways that counteraction can be created?

a. Restraint,

b. Maintaince of counterweight

c. Elevation of body part closet to the weight.

d. Proper position & body alignment

695

8. Failure to maintain correct placement of the patient in bed while he is in traction can result in: distortion in desired result

695

9. Cite five nursing measures that can prevent pressure areas in patients who are bedfast and in various types of traction.

a. Keep linen smooth and tight

b. Used eggcrate or sheepskin onder bony paemises

c. Eliminate any crumbs or other irritating objects from under body part

d. Frequently inspection & cleansing of susceptible body area

e. Apply tincture Benzoin

701

10. What is meant by plaster traction?

To promote continued traction and mobilization a cast is applied over a skeletal traction pin

701

11. External immobilization of a body part can be accomplished by the application of a cast, which allows greater mobility for the patient. What does the typical cast consist of?

Plaster Paris
- impregnated crinoline bandage
- Fiber glass
- stockinette

704

12. How often must a child have a cast changed?

- It depends on the growth spruts.
- Condition of the cast
- Progression of desired condition

708

13. List at least six significant signs and symptoms you would look for when checking a new long leg cast.

a. Pallor
b. Edema
c. Puffiness
d. Purple tint
e. Pressure response delay
f. Pulselessness

708

14. Describe the blanching sign. Pressure is made on nail beds to blanch area, when pressure is release the normal color should return less than 3 seconds

707 15. If a new cast is stained with blood, how can you monitor the amount of bleeding?

Circle the drainage time it initial and check it often

708 16. How often should a patient in a body cast be turned? *2-3 hours*

712 17. What is the purpose of a brace? *To furnish support, provide strength and maintain of body part.*

713 18. How would you measure a patient for standard-type crutches?

16 inches from patients height

713 19. When a patient uses crutches, he or she should know that the weight of the body should be borne by the *Hands .*

> Five-year-old Johnny is being placed in a hip spica cast and will be returned to his unit soon.

704 20. What supplies might you need to prepare the unit for his return? (Name five.)

a. *Bed board to prevent mattress from sagging*
b. *A fracture pan*
c. *Urine - collecting bag to protect cast.*
d. *Cast drier or well - ventilated room*
e. *Possibly an overhead bar and tapeze attched to*

705 21. How long will it probably take for his cast to dry? *24 hrs*

705 22. How can you tell when his cast is dry? *When a chalky white finish*

705-706 23. How can you prevent the rough surface of Johnny's cast from injuring tissues?

By petalling the edges of the cast

706   24. Define the process called *petaling*. _application of water repellant adhesive strip cut to fit around the perineal edge and other rough edges_

706   25. Several days later, when Johnny's mother is preparing to take him home, she asks you what to do when the cast becomes soiled. How would you reply?

Cast can be cleaned with damp cloth c̄ some type of white cleanser. Fast drying white shoe polish

693   26. Traction or methods of exerting pull are used to do all of the following *EXCEPT*:
   a. Compress a part
   b. Prevent a contracture
   c. Relieve muscle spasms
   d. Reduce a dislocated hip

698   27. A skin area that should be particularly checked when Buck's extension is employed is the:
   a. Sacrum
   b. Scapula
   c. Ankle
   d. Heel

696   28. The traction often used in the treatment of a fractured femur in the infant is:
   a. Russell's
   b. Bryant's
   c. A Thomas splint
   d. Buck's extension

704   29. How often a child must have the cast changed depends on all of the following *EXCEPT*:
   a. Rate of growth
   b. Age
   c. Condition of the cast
   d. Progress of the desired correction

697   30. Ninety-degree–ninety-degree traction commonly is used to reduce a fractured femur. Which one of the following is a major nursing consideration in the management of the child in a ninety- degree–ninety-degree traction?
   a. Avoid any movement of bed or traction setup
   b. Maintain proper alignment with the patient flat
   c. Avoid skin breakdown around ankles and heels
   d. Report immediately any signs of restlessness

698   31. Which one of the following types of traction might be ordered to relieve lower back pain?
       a. Balanced traction
       b. Russell's traction
       c. Pelvic traction
       d. Skeletal traction

708   32. A newly casted extremity can suffer impaired circulation. Which one of the following is *not* a sign of a neurovascular complication?
       a. Puffiness
       b. Pallor
       c. Pulselessness
       d. Posturing

709   33. The child who is immobilized because of a fracture needs meticulous skin care, as well as special attention to the diet. Which of the following diets is most appropriate with a liberal fluid intake?
       a. High caloric
       b. High protein
       c. High carbohydrate
       d. High fiber

STUDENT'S NAME _____

Respiratory and Cardiovascular Problems

age Reference

715-716

1. Match the terms on the right with the descriptions on the left.

____b___ Absence of breathing

____d___ Difficult breathing

____e___ Normal breathing

____a___ Abnormal narrowing of a passage or opening

____f___ Collection of pus in a body cavity

____g___ Abnormal dilation and loss of elasticity of the microscopic air sacs

____c___ Excessive amount of fluid within the body tissue

a. Stenosis
b. Apnea
c. Edema
d. Dyspnea
e. Eupnea
f. Empyema
g. Emphysema

2. List the common infectious pneumonias in infants and children under the two major headings

717
a. Bacterial (list four)

(1) Streptococcal

(2) Staphococcal

(3) Pnemoniococcal

(4) H. Infleunze

717
b. Nonbacterial (list two)

(1) Viral

(2) Mycoplasma

251

717

3. Four classic signs and symptoms of pneumonia are:

   a. _anorexia_   c. _listlessness_

   b. _fever_   d. _cough_

717

4. Describe the type of respirations commonly seen in young children with pneumonia.

   Rapid shallow, grunting

   flaring of the nose & retractions

717

5. Two grave signs associated with pneumonia in infants are:

   a. _Cyanosis_

   b. _Rapid weak pulse_

718

6. What three laboratory studies are most helpful in the diagnosis of pneumonia?

   a. _CBC c̄ a diff_

   b. _Tracheal cultures_

   c. _X-Ray film_

717

7. The most common type of pneumonia encountered in infants is: _____

   Pnuemoncoccol

717

8. Penicillin is specific for what type of pneumonia? _Pnuemonococco)_

720

9. Infants who are under 6 months of age and have pneumonia are always hospitalized. List four reasons that would require hospitalization of an older child with pneumonia.

   a. _Unable to take fluids_

   b. _Need oxygen therapy_

   c. _Family not able to take care of child_

   d. _Surgical drainage indicated_

739

10. Label the parts of the normal heart shown in Fig. 34-1.

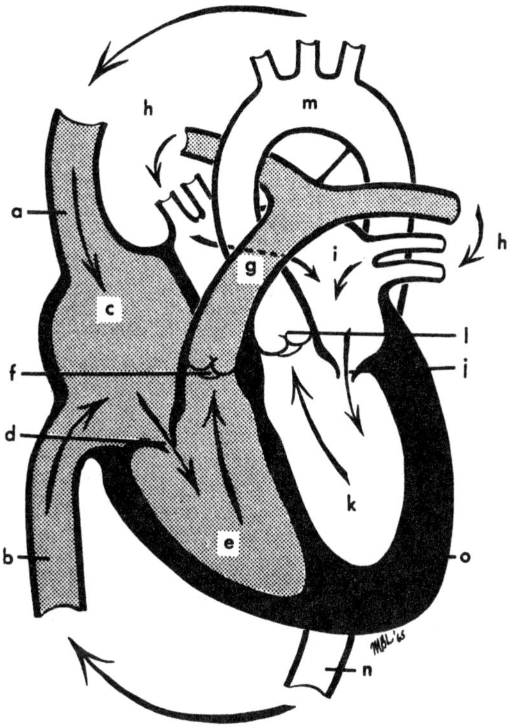

a. _____
b. _____
c. _____
d. _____
e. _____
f. _____
g. _____
h. _____
i. _____
j. _____
k. _____
l. _____
m. _____
n. _____
o. _____

Fig. 34-1. Normal heart and circulation pattern.

741   11. Congenital heart disease refers to a structural abnormality or defect present in the heart at birth. Such a defect creates three problems related to blood flow within the heart and circulation. Define each of the following problems.

a. Volume overload ___more blood than normal enter the ventricle___

b. Pressure overload ___out flow of blood is impeding or slowed___

c. Desaturation ___low saturating circulation in the arterial blood___

741   12. Poor oxygenation in infants often results in ___acidosis___ and ___cyanosis___.

741   13. Define the following common signs and symptoms in the infant with serious congenital heart disease.
a. Cyanosis ___manifestation of blusih lips, nail beds and micsal surface___

b. Tachypnea _Symptoms of flaring nostrils_
Premature, more than 60 per minute

c. Tachycardia _heart rate greater than_
160 beats per minute

d. Effort intolerance _Chiefly manifested by feeding_
problems; infant becomes easily fatigue

e. Failure to thrive _failure to gain weight_

f. Murmur _abnormal heart sounds_

741   14. What specific complication of congenital heart disease warrants prompt cardiac consultation? _Congestive heart failure_

739   15. Match the definitions in the right column with the terms in the left column.

_d_ Echocardiography

_b_ X-ray examination

_e_ Phonocardiography

_c_ Electrocardiography

_a_ Angiography

a. Injection of a contrast medium into the circulation and observation of its flow
b. Permanent recording of the size and shape of the heart
c. Measurements of the electrical activity of the heart
d. Sonar recordings
e. External pulse and heart sound recordings

740   16. Cardiac catheterization is a valid diagnostic procedure used to confirm heart defects. What general information does it reveal? _Pressure in various areas of the cardiocirculatory system._

742   17. When does the ductus arteriosus normally close? _Soon after birth, within a few weeks_

742   18. What are the consequences of a large PDA? *Patentus Ductus arteriosus.* abnormal work load on the left left ventricle ↑ B/P in pulmonary circulation

744   19. Name the three great vessels that sprout from the aortic arch.
- a. Left carotid
- b. Left Sub clavian
- c. Innominate

744   20. Define coarctation. narrowing of the aorta

744   21. How does coarctation affect the pulses of the lower extremities? Pulse are weak and absent

744   22. List four specific complaints of older children with coarctation.
- a. Head ache
- b. Leg cramps
- c. Frequent nosebleeds
- d. Possible excessive fatigue

744   23. What is the definitive treatment for coarctation?
Narrowing protion cut out & rejoined prothesis - pig value — surgery

742   24. What type of problem related to blood flow within the heart does atrial septal defect (ASD) create? Volume overload

742   25. If the pulmonary artery valve is also stenosed, what additional blood flow disturbance occurs? Left to right shunt is reversed, cynotic condition result.

742   26. What three physical problems may the child with an ASD demonstrate?

a. _Decreased resistance to infections_

b. _Lower excercised tolerance_

c. _Physical under development_

742   27. Open heart surgery is usually done to close a large ASD. Can this defect be closed merely by suturing? Explain.

Yes. If the opening is small

742   28. How serious is ventricular septal defect (VSD)?

Depends on the position and size of the defect and the presence of any abnormalities in the heart or great vessels

742   29. When a large opening occurs in the membranous portion of the septum, the blood usually travels from the left to the right side of the heart. Is the child cyanotic or acyanotic? _Acyanotic_

742   30. What usually occurs when pulmonary vascular resistance increases? _____

Shunt is reversed, the child becomes cyanotic

742   31. What is the specific treatment for a large VSD in an infant? _Surgical repair by open heart surgery_

742   32. What are the four classic features of tetralogy of Fallot?

a. _Interventricular septal defect,_

b. _Pulmonary stenosis._

c. _Overriding aorta._

d. _Right ventricle hypertrophy_

743   33. Describe the clinical appearance of the moderately to severely affected young child with tetralogy of Fallot.

Child has blue lips Blue nail bed, dusky tinted skin, become more cyantoic on excertion

Ne likely to be small for age

743   34. Define the "hypoxemic spells" that blue babies typically manifest.

respiratory distress causes deep cynosis, loss of consciousness and possible convulsion

743   35. What are the advantages of squatting, a position commonly assumed by the toddler who has tetralogy?

Improves oxygen in upper portion of body and trapping desaturated blood in lower body

743   36. Why is open heart surgery preferred over the Blalock-Taussig or Waterston operation?

Open heart surgery offers change of total correction

> Six-month-old Billy Gray is assigned to your care today. He is isolated and has a diagnosis of staphylococcal pneumonia.

717   37. Billy's mother tells you that he did not have a cold and wonders how he got pneumonia. How would you reply?

_____

_____

_____

_____

717   38. Little Billy's respirations are 60 per minute, and his color is very pale. Why are his respirations so fast?

_____

_____

_____

717   39. Billy is receiving specific antibiotic therapy every 6 hours by intravenous infusion. What antibiotic is specific for staphylococcal pneumonia? _____

Nafcillin sodium or oxacillin sw

717   40. How long must the antibiotic be given to a seriously ill patient such as Billy?

few weeks

717   41. Initially, Billy was given penicillin. Why?

719   42. Supportive care is as important as antibiotic therapy in lessening the severity of Billy's illness. Note the specific nursing interventions for each of Billy's problems listed on the following chart.

Problems	Intervention
Fever 102° F	
Viscid secretions	
Anorexia	
Dyspnea and flaring nostrils	

716
43. Bronchiolitis is an acute viral illness commonly seen in infants. Fortunately the most severe form of the disease lasts only 1 or 2 days and recovery is usually complete within:
a. 3 days
b. 7 days
c. 14 days
d. 21 days

718
44. A very severe chemical pneumonia can be caused by ingestion of:
a. Perfume
b. Lighter fluid
c. Strychnine
d. Vinegar

718
45. Nasopharyngeal cultures are not of great value in diagnosing pneumonia, because pneumococcal, streptococcal, *H. influenzae*, and staphylococcal organisms are:
a. Present only in the lung
b. Not likely to be found in the nose
c. Uncommon in the throat
d. Present in the nasopharynx of healthy children

718
46. Chlamydia pneumonia is tranmitted to the infant during:
a. Pregnancy
b. Labor
c. Birth
d. Breast-feeding

720   47. When a child with pneumonia is treated at home, the most important aspect of care is:
- a. Correct medication
- b. Complete bed rest
- c. Urinary output
- d. Fluid intake

720   48. Cystic fibrosis (CF) is a hereditary disorder in which there is a generalized dysfunction of the exocrine glands. It especially involves the:
- a. Endocrine glands
- b. Sebaceous glands
- c. Mucous glands
- d. Salivary glands

720   49. CF is genetically transmitted by an autosomal recessive gene. If both parents are carriers, the possibilities for inheritance in offspring are:
- a. One child in four will inherit CF
- b. One child in four will be a carrier
- c. All male children will inherit CF
- d. All female children will be carriers

720   50. A small percentage of infants with CF are in the newborn nursery because of the detection of a:
- a. Respiratory tract infection
- b. Low hemoglobin level
- c. Meconium ileus
- d. Protuberant abdomen

723   51. The diet of an older child with CF should include which modification(s)?
- a. Decreased salt intake
- b. An increase in protein and decrease in fat
- c. Increased protein intake
- d. Increased calories and water miscible vitamins

721   52. Infants and children who should especially be evaluated for CF are those who:
- a. Are mentally retarded
- b. Fail to thrive
- c. Have recurrent asthma
- d. Have constipated stool

722   53. Children with CF usually have serious pulmonary involvement that requires chest physiotherapy (CPT). CPT includes all of the following EXCEPT:
- a. Clapping and vibration
- b. Vital signs
- c. Aerosol medications
- d. Antibiotic therapy

725   54. Young women with CF can bear children, but their ability to conceive seems to be less than normal because of:
- a. Abnormal cervical mucus
- b. Inability to ovulate
- c. A poor nutritional state
- d. Severe pulmonary involvements

725 55. Croup is the same as:
   a. Laryngotracheobronchitis
   b. Epiglottitis
   c. Asthma
   d. Bronchiolitis

726 56. The home treatment for croup includes:
   a. Cool mist
   b. Bed rest
   c. High humidity ✓
   d. Aspirin

726 57. Which one of the following is a *serious* sign of acute airway obstruction?
   a. Decreased pulse rate
   b. Fever
   c. Decreased respirations
   d. Severe stridor

727 58. In cases of moderate to severe croup, intermittent positive- pressure breathing is especially helpful with nebulized:
   a. Normal saline solution
   b. Isoetharine hydrochloride (Bronkosol)
   c. Sterile water
   d. Racemic epinephrine

727 59. A bloody or purulent, foul nasal discharge originating from one nostril only should make one suspicious of:
   a. A sinus infection
   b. Infected adenoids
   c. A foreign body
   d. Meningitis

727 60. A condition characterized by acute respiratory distress, high fever, difficulty in swallowing, and drooling is:
   a. Bronchiolitis
   b. Epiglottitis
   c. Laryngotracheobronchitis
   d. Pneumonia

728 61. The most appropriate position for a child with a nosebleed is:
   a. Lying flat
   b. Sitting up
   c. Lying on the right side
   d. Lying on the left side

728 62. Preschool and young school-age children average how many colds per year?
   a. 2
   b. 6
   c. 10
   d. 12

728

63. Infants should especially be protected from colds because they are affected more seriously than older children. Common problems in the infant include all of the following *EXCEPT*:
    a. Fever
    b. Earaches
    c. Anorexia
    d. Pharyngitis ✓

729

64. Inflammation of the middle ear is a common problem in children. It is related to malfunction of the:
    a. Sinuses
    b. Tympanic membrane
    c. Eustachian tube
    d. Tonsils

729

65. The severe pain associated with otitis media is a result of:
    a. Fluid in the middle ear
    b. Ringing in the ear
    c. Nasal obstruction
    d. Increased temperatures

729

66. Prompt antibiotic therapy is the treatment of choice for acute otitis media. When treatment is delayed, which of the following complications can occur?
    a. Seizures
    b. Brain abscess
    c. Eardrum perforation ✓
    d. Mental retardation

730

67. The nurse should counsel the parent that antibiotic therapy for otitis media should be given for a period of 10 days and that a follow-up visit is necessary in:
    a. 10 days
    b. 3 weeks
    c. 1 month
    d. 2 months

730

68. A common and important residual complication of serous otitis media is:
    a. Pneumonia
    b. Tonsillitis
    c. Laryngotracheobronchitis
    d. Hearing loss

732

69. The best results from tonsillectomy are obtained when the symptoms have been clearly referred to the:
    a. Chest
    b. Neck
    c. Nose
    d. Tonsils

732

70. If bleeding occurs following a tonsillectomy, it usually occurs:
    a. Within 1 week
    b. During the first day
    c. Within the first 3 days
    d. Within a month

732

71. To soothe a sore throat or cough following tonsillectomy, Jane's mother is best counseled to give 5-year-old Jane:
    a. Clear fluids
    b. Ginger ale
    c. Ice cream
    d. Aspirin

734

72. Penicillin is given to children with Group A beta-hemolytic streptococcal pharyngitis for the specific purpose of:
    a. Preventing rheumatic fever
    b. Preventing hepatitis
    c. Easing the painful pharyngitis
    d. Preventing meningitis

736

73. The most effective drug in counteracting bronchospasm in status asthmaticus is:
    a. Epinephrine
    b. Aminophylline
    c. Terfenadine (Seldane)
    d. Pseudoephedrine (Drixoral)

735   74. Asthma is characterized by difficulty in breathing as the result of all of the following *EXCEPT*:
       a. Bronchial spasm   c. Bronchial wheezing ✓
       b. Bronchial edema   d. Bronchial secretions

748   75. A decrease in heart and respiratory rate in infants with congestive heart failure is accomplished by digitalization. A digitalizing dose is usually given over a period of:
       a. 12 hours   c. 24 hours
       b. 16 hours   d. 48 hours

748   76. A maintenance dose of 10% of the digitalizing dosage is usually given every 12 hours but should be withheld when:
       a. The apical pulse is under 100
       b. The patient is sleeping
       c. The patient is scheduled for x-ray examinations
       d. The respirations are over 40

748   77. Signs and symptoms of digoxin (Lanoxin) toxicity include all of the following *EXCEPT*:
       a. Anorexia   c. Bradycardia
       b. Irregular pulse   d. Tachycardia ✓

748   78. Which one of the following nursing measures *does not help* to comfort or to conserve the energy of infants with congestive heart failure:
       a. A sitting position   c. Uninterrupted sleep
       b. Routine feedings   d. Humidified oxygen

748   79. Pulmonary congestion associated with heart failure is characterized by:
       a. Weight gain   c. Weight loss
       b. Vomiting   d. Tachypnea

748   80. Congestion of blood in the systemic venous system can cause:
       a. Enlargement of the spleen   c. Enlargement of the liver
       b. Wheezing   d. Dyspnea

748   81. Damage to cardiac tissue may set the stage for an inflammation of the lining of the heart, which is known as:
       a. Endarteritis   c. Myocarditis
       b. Endocarditis   d. Pericarditis

749   82. The risk of cerebral thrombosis can be reduced in children who have an excess of circulating red blood cells by:
       a. Conserving their energy   c. Administration of digoxin
       b. Frequent blood counts   d. Adequate fluid intake

750   83. The most important feature of rheumatic fever is:
       a. Polyarthralgia   c. Carditis ✓
       b. Polyarthritis   d. Chorea

750   84. Which one of the following is not a major manifestation of rheumatic fever?
       a. Chorea   c. Polyarthritis
       b. Erythema marginatum   d. Positive throat culture ✓

751   85. Children with rheumatic fever must have frequent pulse counts taken. To determine the quality and rhythm of the pulse rate, the nurse must always count for:
a. 30 seconds
b. 1 minute
c. 2 minutes
d. 3 minutes

750   86. A laboratory test that indicates the presence of an inflammatory process in the body is:
a. Blood urea nitrogen
b. Erythrocyte count
c. Sedimentation rate
d. Anti streptolysin O

750   87. A feature of rheumatic fever that is characterized by involuntary muscular twitching is:
a. Sydenham's chorea ✓
b. Blanching sign
c. Cerebral palsy
d. Gower's sign

750   88. The highly distinctive rash of rheumatic fever is called:
a. Erythroderma
b. Erythema infectiosum
c. Erysipelas
d. Erythema marginatum

751   89. The medication that is administered to eliminate any lingering streptococci and to prevent a reinfection of RH is:
a. Sulfonamide
b. Penicillin ✓
c. Prednisone
d. Aspirin

748   90. Clinical manifestations of heart failure in infants include all but one of the following:
a. Tachycardia
b. Dyspnea
c. Hypertension ✓
d. Hepatomegaly

748   91. Edema in infants with CHF is often best demonstrated by:
a. Enlarged spleen
b. Rapid pulse
c. Enlarged liver
d. Weight gain ✓

748   92. Blood-tinged froth and coughing is usually present with which of the following conditions?
a. Pulmonary congestion
b. Acute viral pericarditis
c. System congestion
d. Subacute bacterial endocarditis

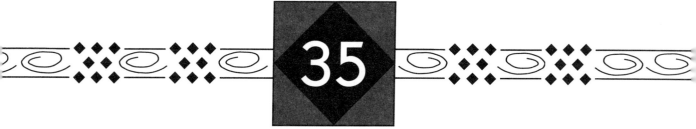

Gastrointestinal and Metabolic Problems

Page Reference

757   1. How does mechanical digestion differ from chemical digestion?

757   2. List six common manifestations of digestive system disorders.

   a. _____

   b. _____

   c. _____

   d. _____

   e. _____

   f. _____

757   3. A common problem associated with long-term administration of antibiotics is thrush. Why?

768   4. Is insulin-dependent diabetes mellitus (IDDM-1) hereditary? _____

768   5. What are two main differences between the child with diabetes and the adult with diabetes?

    a. _____

    _____

    b. _____

    _____

768   6. How is diabetes diagnosed in the child?

768   7. Match the conditions in the left column with the definitions at the right.

    _____ Hyperglycemia

    _____ Glycosuria

    _____ Polydipsia

    _____ Polyuria

    _____ Polyphagia

    _____ Aglycosuria

    _____ Hypoglycemia

    a. Sugar-free urine
    b. Exceptional appetite
    c. Excessive thirst
    d. Increased urinary output
    e. Elevated blood glucose level
    f. Low blood glucose level
    g. Glucose in urine

770-771   8. Compare the nutritional intake of a child with diabetes with that of a healthy non-diabetic child.

771   9. Total calories should be adjusted to meet the individual child's needs. List six factors that must be considered when planning caloric intake.

a. _____

b. _____

c. _____

d. _____

e. _____

f. _____

10. The American Diabetic Association has prepared several recommendations for the calculation of food intake.

770   a. In general, what kind of food does it recommend? _____

_____

771   b. Where should emphasis be placed? _____

_____

769   11. Complete the following chart.

TYPES OF INSULIN			
Type	Onset of action	Peak action (hours after injection)	Effective duration in hours
Regular			
Semilente			
Globin			
NPH			
Lente			

769   12. When both rapid-acting and intermediate-acting insulin are prescribed together, how should they be drawn into the syringe?

769   13. Define "regular insulin coverage."

770   14. List the clinical manifestations of hyperglycemia.

770   15. List the clinical manifestations of hypoglycemia.

772   16. What is glucagon?

773   17. Because the type and dosage of insulin must be individualized for each child, all diabetic regimens must use blood glucose tests to serve as the guide for assessing the levels of control.

                 a. How would you teach 10-year-old Cindy to collect her blood specimen and test it for glucose?

                 b. When and how often should the child check her blood glucose?

> You have been assigned to care for Oscar Little, who is 4 weeks old, weighs 8 lb 4 oz, and has been admitted to the pediatric unit with a diagnosis of pyloric stenosis. His parents tell you that he has been vomiting all of his feedings for the past week. Mrs. Little states that although he has not lost any weight, he has not gained since his 3-week baby check. Despite the frequent vomiting, the baby continues to have a good appetite and takes fluids when they are offered.

758

18. Mrs. Little asks you if all babies with pyloric stenosis have a good appetite. You explain that:

758

19. Most babies with pyloric stenosis lose weight. Why has Oscar not lost weight?

759

20. Describe the Fredet-Ramstedt operation that Oscar will undergo.

759

21. Mrs. Little asks how long Oscar will be in the hospital after his operation. How do you reply?

Leslie White is 2 months old and weighs 6 lb. She has just been admitted to the pediatric unit and placed in an Isolette. Her diagnosis is unknown, but she was admitted because of bloody diarrhea. The doctor asks you to carefully assess the infant's bowel movements while you are caring for her today. During the morning Leslie passes 5 grossly bloody stools that contain large amounts of mucus. You also note that she is very irritable and cries out often. When you report these findings to the physician he tells you that this is exactly what Mrs. White stated in the history and that he suspects that the infant has an intussusception.

760

22. What is intussusception? _____

_____

_____

Mrs. White asks the physician what he plans to do for her infant. The physician explains the nature of the child's condition and tells her that Leslie will be taken to the x-ray film department for a barium enema. He also states that some infants get better after the enema.

760

23. When the physician leaves, Mrs. White tearfully looks to you and asks how a barium enema can help her baby. How would you reply?

757

24. The treatment for esophageal stenosis may include all of the following *EXCEPT*:
    a. Dilations
    b. Tracheotomy
    c. Gastrostomy
    d. Surgical repair

757

25. Thrush and other manifestations of *Candida albicans* associated with prolonged use of antibiotics will resolve when:
    a. Proper mouth hygiene is used
    b. Buttermilk is added to the diet
    c. The drug is discontinued
    d. Nystatin oral suspension is prescribed

757

26. Infants with pyloric stenosis usually manifest symptoms after age:
    a. 2 weeks
    b. 2 months
    c. 3 months
    d. 6 months

759   27. A structural remnant from embryonic life is the persistence of a pouch in the ileum called:
         a. The appendix
         b. Meckel's diverticulum
         c. Wilms' tumor
         d. A cord hernia

759   28. Obstruction of the small intestine, which affects infants and toddlers, may be caused by:
         a. Hirschsprung's disease
         b. Meconium ileus
         c. Intussusception
         d. Appendicitis

761   29. Acute abdominal pain is associated with the symptom colic. Typically the infant cries out and:
         a. Draws up the legs to the abdomen
         b. Stretches out the legs
         c. Hyperextends the head
         d. Stretches out the fingers

761   30. Colic can be caused by the presence of excessive gas in the digestive tract, which can be prevented by:
         a. An increase of carbohydrates in the formula
         b. The use of plastic nursing bottles
         c. Careful bubbling after feedings
         d. The use of nipples with small holes

761   31. Diarrheal disease of infancy is a syndrome, the course of which varies with all of the following *EXCEPT*:
         a. Age
         b. Size
         c. Cause
         d. Race

761   32. Most acute diarrheas appear to be caused by:
         a. Anatomical abnormalities
         b. Viruses
         c. Emotions
         d. Malabsorption syndromes

762   33. When a misplaced loop of intestine becomes trapped in an inguinal hernia, the hernia is described as:
         a. Strangulated
         b. Doubled
         c. Incarcerated
         d. Gangrenous

763   34. Umbilical hernias often close spontaneously after:
         a. Age 4 years
         b. The umbilicus heals
         c. The child learns to walk
         d. Puberty

764

35. Ingested pinworm eggs are hatched in the:
    a. Esophagus
    b. Stomach
    c. Intestine
    d. Anus

766

36. Which of the following is the most common cause of chronic diarrhea in children past the age of 2 years?
    a. *Giardia lamblia*
    b. *Ascaris lumbricoides*
    c. *Enterobius vermicularis*
    d. *Escherichia coli*

766

37. Suspected cases of giardiasis are diagnosed by collecting daily stool specimens for how many days?
    a. 1 day
    b. 2 days
    c. 3 days
    d. 4 days

774

38. In order to avoid hypoglycemia, blood glucose measurements should not be less than:
    a. 70 mg/dl
    b. 80 mg/dl
    c. 90 mg/dl
    d. 100 mg/dl

Genitourinary Problems

Page Reference

780

1. To better understand pathology of the urinary system, review the anatomy involved by labeling Fig. 36-1 as indicated.

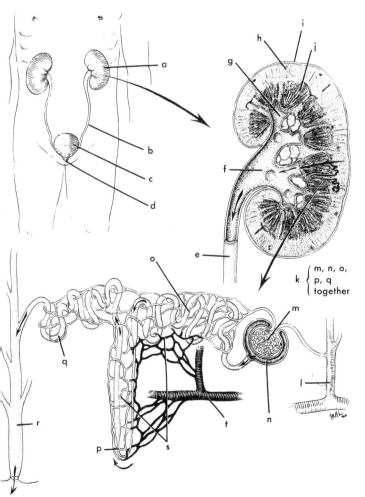

Fig. 36-1.

a. _____

b. _____

c. _____

d. _____

e. _____

f. _____

g. _____

h. _____

i. _____

j. _____

k. _____

l. _____

m. _____

n. _____

o. _____

p. _____

q. _____

r. _____

s. _____

t. _____

781

2. The three basic processes involved in the production of urine are:

a. Filtration — _____

b. Reap' — _____

c. Sect' — _____

779-781

3. Match the term with the appropriate definitive phrase.

_____ Reflux
_____ Uremia
_____ Hematuria
_____ Oliguria
_____ Enuresis
_____ Albuminuria
_____ Polyuria

a. Excessive urine output
b. Retention of nitrogenous products in the blood
c. A backward flow
d. Albumin in the urine
e. Blood in the urine
f. Scanty urine output
g. Bed-wetting when urinary control should be present

4. Cryptorchidism, or undescended testicle, is important to treat for cosmetic and psychological reasons.

785

a. Three other reasons for recommending treatment include:

(1) _____

(2) _____

(3) _____

786

b. Name two ways that cryptorchidism can be treated.

(1) _____

(2) _____

> Fifteen-month-old Peter Green has been admitted to the hospital for a hypospadias repair.

784

5. Define hypospadias, and why was Peter scheduled for surgery at his young age.

784

6. After Peter's urethroplasty, what nursing care and observation directly related to his surgical repair should you expect? (Name three considerations.)

a. _____

b. _____

c. _____

784

7. Peter has had a severe type of hypospadias. Will there be any indication of his childhood surgery in later years?

> Three-year-old Esther Collins recently has had several severe urinary tract infections. She has not responded well to antibiotic therapy and is not her usual lively, good-natured self. Her physician, Dr. Plumb, wants to investigate further to try to discover any underlying reasons for her difficulty. Esther is admitted to the hospital for a cystoscopy, voiding cystourethrogram, and a renal ultrasound.

787

8. For what two types of problems is Dr. Plumb searching?

    a. _____

    b. _____

787

9. As the result of her diagnostic tests results, Esther is scheduled for surgery and a ureteral reimplantation. How does this procedure aid a patient with a history of recurrent urinary tract infection?

787

10. When Esther returns from surgery, she has three draining urinary catheters: a suprapubic and two ureteral catheters. Where do these tubes originate, and what are their purposes?

787

11. You are assigned to assist with Esther postoperative care. List four important nursing considerations involving this specific surgery.

    a. _____

    b. _____

    c. _____

    d. _____

787

12. Because of the prompt treatment of her underlying urinary disorder, Esther's

    prognosis should be: _____

> Tommy Tucker was getting fat—at least that is what his mother first thought as she struggled to get his blue corduroy trousers over his plump tummy. Even his face looked different. His eyes were a bit swollen. Over the last few weeks Tommy had changed in a number of ways. He was tired, irritable, and quite pale. He had had frequent colds during the winter. As Mrs. Tucker thought about all this, she decided that it was time to take her listless 4-year-old son for a physical checkup.

791

13. Tommy had his physical examination. After Tommy's laboratory results were available, the doctor sat down and talked to Mrs. Tucker about a condition he called the *nephrotic syndrome*. On his recommendation Tommy was admitted to the hospital the following day. What three laboratory findings probably pointed to the diagnosis?

    a. _____

    b. _____

    c. _____

791-792

14. You have the responsibility of Tommy's care the next morning. What type of procedures or observations should you expect to be included in his nursing care plan? (List six.)

    a. _____

    b. _____

    c. _____

    d. _____

    e. _____

    f. _____

> Your next door neighbor, Billy Blake, is terribly disappointed. He tells you that his best friend just asked him to stay all night at his house on Halloween, but Billy knows he cannot go. His folks will not allow him, not until he learns not to wet the bed. After all, they reason, an 8-year-old should know better. You ask Billy if his parents have ever asked a doctor about the problem. He says he does not know. You do a lot of babysitting for the Blake family.

793   15. What might you suggest to Billy's parents regarding the problem?

779   16. The nephron, the functional unit of the kidney:
         a. Removes toxic metabolic wastes and excessive nontoxic substances from the blood
         b. Absorbs secretions, such as creatinine, ammonia, and certain drugs from the blood
         c. Normally filters both water and sugar through its glomerulus
         d. Normally filters protein and RBCs from the bloodstream

782   17. All of the following are signs or symptoms that may indicate urinary tract problems in the infant *EXCEPT*:
         a. Abdominal enlargement
         b. Frequent voidings
         c. Increased thirst
         d. Febrile seizures

785   18. Cryptorchidism (testicular maldescent) is rarely associated with symptoms, but it is associated with an increased incidence of:
         a. Infection
         b. Enuresis
         c. Injury
         d. Reflux

786   19. The most common cause of urinary tract infection is:
         a. Injury
         b. Viruses
         c. Obstruction
         d. Bacteria

786   20. The most common way in which urinary tract infections occur is via:
         a. The bloodstream
         b. The ascending route (the urethra)
         c. The lymphatics
         d. Trauma

785   21. Which on of the following conditions is a major cause of kidney failures in children?
         a. Hypertension
         b. Chronic glomerulonephritis
         c. Nephrotic syndrome
         d. Acute glomerulonephritis

787   22. Reflux (regurgitation of urine from the bladder into the ureter) is detected by:
         a. Intravenous pyelogram
         b. Cystogram
         c. Cystourethrography
         d. Urinalysis

787   23. When caring for a child with pyelonephritis, the nurse needs to remember that the patient should:
    a. Be isolated because of infectious disease
    b. Have continuous intake and output determinations daily
    c. Have urinalysis and culture checked daily
    d. Have his BP taken twice daily

789   24. Wilms' tumor is one of the most common abdominal neoplasms of childhood. It is a malignancy of the kidney that:
    a. Develops from the adrenal gland
    b. Manifests early signs and symptoms
    c. Responds well to early detection and treatment
    d. Is more common in boys than in girls

789   25. Which of the following medications are most effective in the treatment of Wilms' tumor?
    a. Vincristine and prednisone
    b. Vincristine and actinomycin D
    c. Actinomycin D and methotrexate
    d. Methotrexate and vincristine

789   26. The most serious and major complicating factor in patients with Wilms' tumor is:
    a. Hemorrhage
    b. Anuria
    c. Metastasis
    d. Shock

790   27. The nephrotic syndrome is a chronic, intermittent renal condition characterized by all of the following *EXCEPT*:
    a. Anasarca
    b. High serum albumin level
    c. Proteinuria
    d. High serum cholesterol level

792   28. Relapses of the nephrotic syndrome are often associated with urinary tract infections and:
    a. Anemia
    b. Respiratory tract infections
    c. Dehydration
    d. Hypotension

794   29. Torsion of the testis can occur at any time and is associated with:
    a. Fever
    b. Hematuria
    c. Anuria
    d. Severe pain

794   30. A complete evaluation of the child with enuresis should include all of the following *EXCEPT*:
    a. Careful medical history
    b. Physical examination
    c. Diet analysis
    d. Urine culture

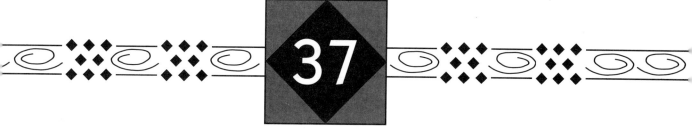

Hematological Problems

Page Reference

800   1. What is the name given to a condition in which the total hemoglobin content of the blood is abnormally reduced? _____Anemia_____

800   2. What is the substance in red blood cells that is necessary for the normal transport of oxygen to the body cells? _____hemogoblin_____ .

800   3. List three causes of iron-deficiency anemia.

  a. _Acute or chronic blood loss_

  b. _Dietary deficiency of iron_

  c. _Impaired absorption of iron_

800   4. List four common clinical manifestations of iron-deficiency anemia.

  a. _listlessness_

  b. _Anorexia_

  c. _Irritability_

  d. _Pallor of the mucus membrane_

800   5. Sickle cell disease (SCD) is found primarily in which group of people in the United states?
        _____African - American_____

800   6. The sickling abnormality is responsible for the synthesis of a different type of hemoglobin. What is the cause of the defect in SCD?
        One amino acid of the 574 that make up normal hemoglobin.

802   7. The sickle cell trait (SCT) confers some degree of protection against the lethal effects of what disease?

malaria

802   8. When the blood of the one parent shows the SCT and the child has SCD, what condition may be present in the other parent?

Thalassemia

805   9. Classic hemophilia is the result of a defect in a gene on which chromosome?

_X_

805   10. The defect in clot formation causing classic hemophilia is due to lack of:

Factor   V-III

807   11. Define leukemia (ALL).

a primary malignant disease of the bone marrow characterized by an abnormal increase of immature white blood cell or undifferentiated blast cells

807   12. How does leukemia affect development of normal blood cells?

By the uncontrolled proliferation which leads to Anemia, infection & bleeding

807   13. Leukemia is suspected when immature WBCs are found in the circulation. What particular test is necessary for the unequivocal diagnosis of leukemia?

Bone marrow aspiration analysis

807   14. The lowest incidence of leukemia is found in what group of American children?

Non white children

807   15. List five clinical manifestations of leukemia.

a. _fever_

b. _fatigue_

c. _weight loss_

d. _pallor_

e. _bruises_

809   16. Chemotherapy is the mainstay of treatment of leukemia. What is the objective of chemotherapy?

A complete remission

808   17. Toxicity manifested by bone marrow depression can result from use of any of the antileukemic drugs. What are the clinical manifestations of bone marrow depression?

a. _Anemia_

b. _Leukopenia_

c. _Thrombocytopenia_

811   18. The best prognostic indication of the length of survival of children with acute leukemia is:

The length of first remission, the longer the remission endures the better the prognosis.

Five-year-old Debra Wells is on her way to the pediatric unit with her mother. She has had a bone marrow aspiration performed in the clinic and is now being admitted with a diagnosis of acute lymphocytic leukemia (ALL). Debra will receive intrathecal (spinal) injections of methotrexate during the course of her induction therapy.

---

809   19. Why will Debra receive intrathecal injections of methotrexate?

_____

_____

_____

811-812   20. While Debra is undressing, her mother asks you about remissions. She wants to know if all children have remissions. She also wants to know how long a remission lasts and how she will know when it is over. How would you respond?

_____

_____

_____

_____

800   21. The major cause of iron-deficiency anemia in infants is:
a. Excessive growth spurt
b. Inadequate iron supply at birth
c. Insufficient dietary intake of iron
d. Impaired absorption of iron

800   22. Low hemoglobin concentrations indicate iron-deficiency anemia. Suggestive laboratory values that indicate this condition are:
- a. Less than 14 g/dl
- b. Less than 13 g/dl
- c. Less than 12 g/dl
- d. Less than 11 g/dl

803   23. Children with sickle cell disease often have a severe degree of anemia that occurs as a result of intravascular sickling. This condition is associated with which one of the following?
- a. Infection
- b. Over hydration
- c. Fetal hemoglobin
- d. Immobilization

805   24. In most healthy children, the average antihemophilic globulin (factor VIII) level is about 100%. In mildly hemophilic patients factor VIII levels are:
- a. Less than 1%
- b. 2% to 5%
- c. 5% to 10%
- d. 10% to 20%

806   25. Factor VIII concentrate can be given in any amount to control hemorrhage in these patients. However, the nurse must remember that factor VIII falls to half its original strength in:
- a. 1 hour
- b. 4 to 6 hours
- c. 8 to 10 hours
- d. 24 hours

806   26. The precise level of factor VIII needed to control bleeding is unknown but the amount of factor VIII should be related to the:
- a. Age of the patient
- b. Seriousness of the bleeding
- c. Size of the patient
- d. Amount available

812   27. Idiopathic thrombocytopenic purpura is a syndrome characterized by bruises, purpura, and petechia resulting from a greatly:
- a. Increased platelet count
- b. Decreased RBC count
- c. Increased RBC count
- d. Decreased platelet count

813   28. A major complication of idiopathic thrombocytopenic purpura, especially in the early course of the condition, is:
- a. Intracranial edema
- b. Infection
- c. Intracranial hemorrhage
- d. Blindness

807

29. The diagnosis of acute lymphocytic leukemia (ALL) is suspected when the child initially has which one of the following?
   a. Fever associated with infection
   b. Chronic iron-deficiency anemia
   c. Nasal bleeding after injury
   d. Immature WBCs in circulating blood

809

30. Initial treatment of ALL consists of intermittent high doses of several drugs in combination plus:
   a. Blood transfusions
   b. Prophylactic CNS therapy
   c. Platelet transfusions
   d. Prophylactic antibiotic therapy

809

31. A complete remission of the disease ALL is characterized by restoration to normal health and which one of the following?
   a. No evidence of pain
   b. Increased red blood cell count
   c. Freedom from infections
   d. Normal labs

811

32. Although most children with ALL can be cured, children of which one of the following subgroups have a very poor prognosis?
   a. B cell leukemia
   b. Children under 10 years of age
   c. Nonwhite children
   d. Siblings of leukemic children

STUDENT'S NAME _____

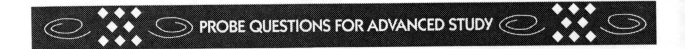

1. Children with cancer experience a great deal of anxiety pertaining to painful procedures such as bone marrow aspirations and lumbar punctures. List and discuss the adverse effects that have been documented to be associated with pain, fear, and anxiety in children with cancer. Should all children be premedicated for painful procedures? How do nurses feel about premedicating children? List three other interventions that are effective in the preparation of children for painful procedures, especially those in the pediatric oncology setting.

REFERENCES

Broome ME: Preparation of children for painful procedures, *Pediatr Nurs* 16(6):537-541, 1990.

Klein ER: Premedicating children for painful invasive procedure, *J Pediatr Oncology Nurs* 9(4):170-179, 1992.

Zeltzer LK et al: Report of the subcommittee on the management of pain associated with procedures in children with cancer, *Pediatrics* 36(5):826-831, 1990.

2. Breast-feeding is best for almost all infants. Discuss the nutritional and immunological superiority of breast milk for nourishing young infants. List three effective techniques for the promotion of breast-feeding. Why are infants who breast-feed more likely to have colic? What is meant by infant "colic"? How closely does formula resemble human milk? Discuss the effects of early formula supplementation on breast-feeding.

REFERENCES

Cervisi J et al: Office management of the infant with colic, *J Pediatr Health Care* 5(4):184-190, 1992.

Howard CR and Wsitzman M: Breast or bottle: practical aspects of infant nutrition in the first 6 months, *Pediatr Ann* 21(10):619-631, 1992.

Kurinij N and Shiono PH: Early formula supplementation of breast-feeding, *Pediatrics* 88(4):745-750, 1991.

NAPNAP Position Statement on Breast-feeding, *J Pediatr Health Care* 7(6):289, 1993.

3. Physiological jaundice is commonly encountered in the newborn. When does physiological jaundice first appear and why? Is it more common in breast-fed babies or formula-fed babies? Discuss the management of physiological jaundice. Give two major causes of pathological jaundice in the newborn. Discuss the indications for liver transplant following the Kasai operation. What are the major threats to the transplant recipient?

REFERENCES

Buzby M: Assessment of hyperbilirubinemia in full-term infants. Part II, *J Pediatr Health Care* 5(4):210-212, 1991.

Hicks BA and Altman RP: The jaundiced newborn, *Pediatr Clin North Am* 40(6):1161-1175, 1993.

Newman TB and Maisels MJ: Evaluation and treatment of jaundice in the term newborn: a kinder, gentler approach, *Pediatrics* 89(5):809-818, 1992.

Sokal EM et al: Liver transplantation in children less than 1 year of age, *J Pediatr* 117(2, part 1):205, 1990.

4. Cystic fibrosis (CF) is the most common lethal genetic disease of childhood. What is the likelihood of being a carrier? Discuss the incidence and genetic aspects of CF. Recent developments in DNA technology allow people to know whether they are at risk to have a child with a genetic mutation. Does DNA testing identify the presence of a CF mutation? Discuss the goal of antimicrobial therapy in the management of CF. What is the most feasible system for long-term antimicrobial therapy for patients with CF? What is the current survival rate of children with CF?

REFERENCES

Beaudet AL: Genetic testing for cystic fibrosis, *Pediatr Clin North Am* 39(2):213-228, 1992.

Hammond LJ, Caldwell S, Campbell PW: Cystic fibrosis, intravenous antibiotics and home therapy, *J Pediatr Health Care* 5(1):24-30, 1991.

Hulsebus DR and Williams J: Cystic fibrosis: a new perspective in genetic counseling, *J Pediatr Health Care* 6(6):338-342, 1992.

5. Asthma is responsible for a significant proportion of both acute and chronic illness in childhood. What type of infection often triggers wheezing lower respiratory tract illness in infants and toddlers? What is the pathophysiology of exacerbations of asthma? Discuss the risk of developing a lower respiratory tract illness in infants of mothers who smoke. Is there a genetic basis for wheezing lower respiratory tract illness? Discuss the comprehensive management and educational intervention for children with asthma.

REFERENCES

Excerpts from the NAEP executive summary: guidelines for the diagnosis and management of asthma, *Pediatr Ann* 21(9):537-565, 1992.

Moe EL et al: Implementation of "open airways" as an educational intervention for children with asthma in an HMO, *J Pediatr Health Care* 6(5):251-253, 1992.

Morgan WJ and Martinez FD: Risk factors for developing wheezing and asthma in childhood, *Pediatr Clin North Am* 39(6):1185-1203, 1992.

6. Survivors of serious illness during the neonatal period continue to have ongoing medical and nursing problems. An example of such children are those graduated from the neonatal intensive care unit who have bronchopulmonary dysplasia (BPD). Describe BPD and discuss the problems associated with this condition. Are these children developmentally delayed? Discuss the family's adaptation to prolonged hospitalization and home oxygen management of the infant with severe BPD.

REFERENCES

Goldberg S: Chronic illness and early development, *Pediatr Ann* 19(1):35, 1990.
Goldson E: Bronchopulmonary dysplasia *Pediatr Ann* 19(1)13, 1990.
Klein-Berndt S: Bronchopulmonary dysplasia in the family: a longitudinal case study, *Pediatr Nurs* 17(6):607-611, 1991.

7. The most common conditions that raise questions about the possibility of inflicted injuries are those involving the skin. The age of bruises can be dated by their color and degree of swelling. How old is a bruise that is green? Nonaccidental bruises can appear in the same locations as accidental bruises but are more commonly found in which locations? Bruising on the wrists and ankles results from what kind of inflicted injury? Do infants have self-inflicted bruises? How does bruising in infancy differ from bruising in toddlers?

REFERENCES

Chadwick DL: The diagnosis of inflicted injury in infants and young children, *Pediatr Ann* 21(8)26-32, 1990.
Hyden PW and Gallagher TA: Child abuse interventions in the emergency room, *Pediatr Clin North Am* 39(5):1068-1069, 1992.
Jurgrau A: How to spot child abuse, *RN* 53(10):26-32, 1990.

8. The most important factors influencing the incidence of flame and scald burns (thermal) are age, sex, and economic status. Children less than 5 years of age are the most prone to thermal burns. Describe the "stocking, glove" burn that is characteristic of inflicted injury. Most of the fatal burns are from what type of burn injury? What are the estimated costs of burn injuries to children, and are there differences between pediatric and adult patients? List five methods of reducing the risk of burn injury for children in their care.

REFERENCES

Erikson EJ et al: Differences in mortality from thermal injury between pediatric and adult patients, *J Pediatr Surg* 26(7):821-825, 1991.
Finkelstein JL et al: Pediatric burns, an overview, *Pediatr Clin North Am* 39(5):1145-1163, 1992.
McLaughlin E and Brigham PA: Stop carelessness? No, reduce burn risk, *Pediatr Ann* 21(7):423-428, 1992.

9. What are the four most common disorders causing alopecia in children? What is the difference between alopecia universalis and alopecia areata? Is the course of alopecia areata predictable or unpredictable? Do children with alopecia areata have a regrowth of hair?

REFERENCES

Atton AV and Tunnessen WW Jr: Alopecia in children—the most common causes, *Pediatr Rev* 12(1):25, 1990.
Blum NJ, Barone VJ, Friman PC: A simplified behavioral treatment for trichotillomania: report of two cases, *Pediatrics* 91(5):993-995, 1993.
Castiglia PT: Alopecia, *J Pediatr Health Care* 5(1):44-46, 1991.

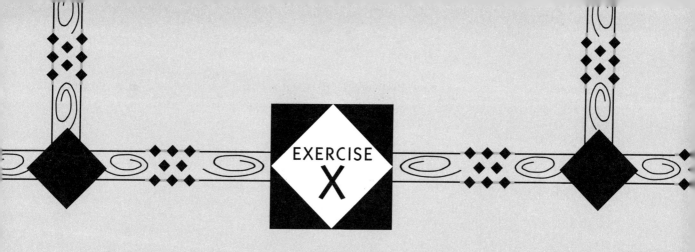

THE CHILD AND FAMILY WITH SPECIAL NEEDS

For most children, the period of hospitalization is brief. However, for a few patients, hospitalization can be very long. The severely ill child who has a long complicated convalescence, the child undergoing elaborate orthopedic corrections or the teenager with a spinal cord injury, are all examples of relatively long-term patients. Many of these children are trying to recapture skills once considered automatic while others are adjusting to new expectations and goals. Although this exercise deals primarily with rehabilitative nursing care, the last section deals with the terminally ill child. Few nursing assignments are more challenging than helping a family and child who has an illness that is often fatal. After reviewing these two chapters, the student will have a better understanding of the need to provide comprehensive professional care and support to the patient and family.

CLINICAL TIE-IN

1. Every hospital that provides a rehabilitation service for children has a rehabilitation team. Who comprises the rehab team in your hospital?
2. How many children on the unit have severe head injuries? How could these injuries have been prevented?
3. What is the policy regarding sibling visitation on the rehab unit?
4. Is there a Ronald McDonald House available to parents near your hospital? To whom is the house available?
5. What is the policy regarding informing a child of his impending death? Who explains this information to the child?
6. What support groups are available to parents who have lost a child?

STUDENT'S NAME ____________________

38

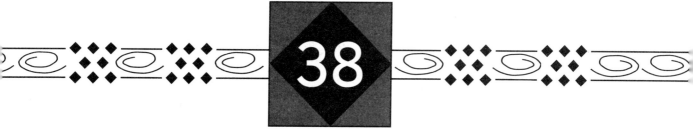

Rehabilitation

Page Reference

817 1. Define the term *habilitation.*

____

____

____

818 2. What is the overall goal of pediatric rehabilitation?

____

____

____

820 3. What three recommendations, important for all hospitalized children, are particularly critical in the rehabilitation setting?

a. ____________________

b. ____________________

c. ____________________

818 4. Ideally, a rehabilitation program provides three interacting therapeutic units. What are they?

a. ____________________

b. ____________________

c. ____________________

Jimmy is a 10-year-old boy who has been transferred to the rehabilitation unit from intensive care. Two days before, he was involved in an automobile accident. At present he is totally unresponsive but medically stable. He has an indwelling catheter attached to closed urinary drainage. A nasogastric tube is used for high-protein, low-carbohydrate blenderized feedings every 4 hours. Other than a bruise on his forehead, no injuries are apparent.

824-825

5. List at least six possible problems associated with prolonged bed rest and immobility that Jimmy and his nurses might have to face, and indicate one nursing intervention that can prevent or ease each problem.

a. _____

_____

b. _____

_____

c. _____

_____

d. _____

_____

e. _____

_____

f. _____

_____

825

6. Jimmy developed a red area over the left trochanter, even though he was turned every 2 hours. What is the first principle of skin care applicable to this situation?

_____

_____

825

7. The method for relieving pressure from the buttocks of the patient who is wheelchair bound is called "chair raise." What is the recommended frequency for this procedure when the patient is paraplegic?

_____

_____

> Julie is a 15-year-old girl who was injured in the family car when leaving for summer vacation. She has paraplegia at the T5 level and is now mobilized in her own wheelchair.

822

8. Julie has been up in her wheelchair for 4 hours. She is now perspiring and complains of feeling warm and having a headache. What should be your first action?

   What condition might these symptoms indicate? _____

   _____

   _____

818-821

9. Julie is now ready for her first overnight pass experience. She has achieved independence in her skin, bowel, and bladder programs, can dress herself, and can transfer from her wheelchair with minimal assistance. What areas of the home do you think might pose problems to her independence? Give two examples.

   a. _____

   b. _____

820

10. While she was at home Julie's father asked her to try to move her toes. When she could not, he stated, "You're not trying; you can if you want to." What psychological stage of parental mourning might this illustrate? If you were present, what might you have said?

Tom is a 15-year-old who suffered a spinal cord injury at the T10 level from a gunshot wound 3 months ago. He has a complete loss of sensation and paralysis below the T10 level. Patients who have undergone such a personal loss experience a sequence of mourning similar to that of bereaved parents.

820

11. Match the statements made by Tom and the descriptions of his behavior on the left with the appropriate stage of mourning on the right. These observations were made over a 3-month period and demonstrate various stages of his progression through the mourning process.

_____ "Why did this happen to me?"

_____ "I know I shouldn't have been fooling around with that gun."

_____ "When are you guys gonna let me out of this bed so I can get walking again?"

_____ Repeatedly pushing his parents to buy him a new surfboard

_____ Complaining about the "rotten care" he has been getting "around this dump"

_____ Refusing to attempt a nighttime proning program after its benefits have been fully explained

_____ Agreeing to visit a school that has modified buildings and an elevator for wheelchair-dependent students

_____ Volunteering to assist with the weekly activities for the younger Cub Scouts on the unit

_____ Repeatedly failing to be on the unit on time for his intermittent catheterizations

a. Shock and denial
b. Developing awareness
c. Restitution

818

12. Pediatric rehabilitation is based on the concepts that each person is unique, possessing individual basic worth, and that:
a. Rehabilitation is less expensive initially than custodial care
b. Rehabilitation should be available for all
c. Rehabilitation is ideally a team endeavor
d. Total independence must be achieved by a person to merit respect

818

13. The overall goal of rehabilitation requires that the skills of communication be employed constantly to ensure:
a. Staff conferences daily
b. A minimum of care
c. Continuity of patient care
d. Monetary resources

818

14. The rehabilitation of disabled children is more complex because of their continued need for:
a. Independence
b. Growth
c. Motivation
d. Education

818   15. Unit staffing on a rehabilitation unit should be _____ above the usual medical-surgical levels:
        a. 10% to 15%
        b. 20% to 30%
        c. 30% to 60%
        d. 70% to 80%

830   16. Older children with spinal cord damage may be taught self- catheterization. All of the following prerequisites for learning clean self-catheterization are necessary *EXCEPT*:
        a. A urologic workup
        b. The ability to tell time
        c. Sensation in the genital area
        d. The use of hands

818   17. To prevent complications and further loss of function, the nurse must initiate the principles of rehabilitation:
        a. At the onset of the injury
        b. After the acute phase of the injury
        c. Before the patient is discharged
        d. After the medical history has been taken

822   18. In dealing with patients with spinal cord injury, the nurse must know that:
        a. Paraplegics have some use of their lower extremities
        b. The higher the cord injury, the more extensive the deficits encountered
        c. Quadriplegia involves sensory deficiencies of the upper extremities only
        d. Excessive perspiration below the level of cord injury is typical

822   19. Common symptoms of autonomic dysreflexia, a complication of spinal cord injury above the T6 level, include:
        a. Sweating and pallor
        b. Tachycardia and hypertension
        c. Hypertension and sweating
        d. Pallor and tachycardia

827   20. Venous pooling and the danger of thrombosis in immobilized patients can be decreased by:
        a. Range of motion exercises
        b. Open-toed support stockings
        c. Frequent monitoring of vital signs
        d. Prolonged use of the sitting position

828   21. The least important aspect of the management of the neurogenic bladder:
        a. Preservation of normal urinary tract anatomy
        b. Prevention of significant urinary infection
        c. Position during clean intermittent catheterization
        d. Attainment of social urinary continence

828   22. Which of the following when injured is least likely to cause neurogenic bladder disease?
        a. Brain
        b. Peripheral nerves
        c. Kidney
        d. Spinal cord

829   23. The most common cause of neurogenic bladder in a young child is:
     a. Hydrocephalus
     b. Meningitis
     c. Spinal cord injury
     d. Myelodysplasia

830   24. Clean intermittent catheterization (CIC) provides a means of protecting the kidney. It generally is performed every:
     a. 2 hours
     b. 4 hours
     c. 6 hours
     d. 8 hours

830   25. During a CIC procedure the catheter is inserted until a stream of urine is obtained. The catheter is then advanced:
     a. 1 inch
     b. 2 inches
     c. 3 inches
     d. 4 inches

830   26. Children at risk for upper urinary tract deterioration can be identified early by regular medical supervision and:
     a. Bed wetting at night
     b. Complete urodynamic studies
     c. Asymptomatic positive urine cultures
     d. Wetting between catheterizations

832   27. A bowel-training program can be difficult or impossible to achieve if:
     a. Meals are irregular
     b. Bananas and cheese are eaten
     c. Physical activity patterns are slowed
     d. A suppository must be given each day

Grief and Loss

Page Reference

838

1. What are the four stages of mourning as described by Bowlby?

    a. _____

    b. _____

    c. _____

    d. _____

Eight-year-old Mark is going to be admitted to the pediatric unit to have a bone marrow aspiration done and to be started on chemotherapy for acute lymphocytic leukemia. When Mark arrives, you will be admitting him and expect to be assigned to his care during the next few days. Mark is the oldest of four children in his family; the others are all girls. To answer any questions he may ask, you should review a child's concept of death and your own attitude about terminal illness and death.

836

2. What factors influence a child's concept of death? List at least two.

    a. _____

    b. _____

836

3. At what age does a child usually achieve a realistic concept of death?_____

508, 511, 512

4. Think back about the specific reason for Mark's hospitalization. How can you help to protect Mark from the fears he might have?

> Mark arrives at the nurses' station at 10 am with his father and mother. His neck glands are very large, and he appears weak and "sick." The charge nurse introduces you to Mark and his parents, Mr. and Mrs. Grey. After a few words of greeting you accompany the family to a four-bed ward where Mark will occupy a bed next to a window. A 6-year-old boy with acute myeloblastic leukemia is in the bed directly across from Mark's unit. The other two beds are empty.

507, 508, 839

5. Mark is staying close to his mother. Should you ask Mark's parents to wait outside while Mark puts on his pajamas? Discuss parental participation in the care of the hospitalized child and of Mark in particular.

839

6. Mrs. Grey asks the physician about Mark's condition. He tells her, "Mark has an infection, too." Mrs. Grey looks at her husband and exclaims, "I told you we should have taken Mark to the doctor last week." Mr. Grey replies softly that it is not all his fault. What do you think is happening?

839

7. What can you do that might help?

837-840
8. When you have completed the recording of the admission procedure, you note that Mark has fallen asleep. His parents are still at his side. The physician asks Mrs. and Mrs. Grey to come to his office. What could you say that would help Mr. and Mrs. Grey to know that Mark will be cared for while they are gone?

837
9. It is time for your lunch, and Mr. and Mrs. Grey are not back yet, but Mark is still asleep. What should you be sure to tell the staff before leaving?

837
10. When you return, Mr. and Mrs. Grey are at the bedside, and Mark is holding his mother's hand. They ask about food for Mark, but you know that he is going to have his bone marrow examination soon. How will you answer their inquiry?

836
11. Children do not have an awareness or understanding of death until about age:
    a. 3 years
    b. 4 years
    c. 5 years
    d. 6 years

836
12. Children seem gradually to be accommodating themselves to the proposition that death is final at about:
    a. 4 years
    b. 6 years
    c. 9 years
    d. 12 years

836   13. Children usually achieve a realistic concept of death by age:
a. 8 years
b. 10 years
c. 12 years
d. 16 years

836   14. Children are equipped with the intellectual tools necessary to comprehend time, space, life, and death in a logical manner as they approach the period of:
a. Preschool
b. School age
c. Puberty
d. Adolescence

837   15. The nurse can best help a child allay his fears by:
a. Helping the parents
b. Talking to the child
c. Holding the child
d. Reading to the child

836   16. Children who are terminally ill rarely manifest an overt concern about death, probably because they:
a. Have been shielded from reality
b. Repress their anxiety about it
c. Do not want to hurt their parents
d. Have been deprived of the opportunity

836   17. A nurse can best help answer the child's questions about death if he/she understands:
a. The child's parents' fears
b. The child's concept of death
c. The mourning process
d. His/her own fears of death

837   18. Young children suffering from terminal illness are subjected to all of the following stresses EXCEPT:
a. Separation from parents
b. Financial
c. Traumatic procedures
d. Isolation

837   19. One of the most important aspects in the management of the child with a terminal illness is:
a. Playing with him
b. Helping his grieving parents
c. Keeping his room quiet
d. Having conferences with the doctor

838   20. Specialized centers for the care of the dying are called:
a. Intensive care units
b. Hospices
c. Special care units
d. Clinics

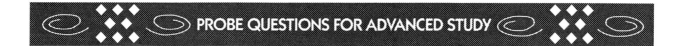

1. The understanding of death is a developmental process. Discuss how children view death at various stages of development. Do children grieve? Is the impact of a death on adolescents less severe than for young children? Discuss the characteristics of nurses who are best equipped to deal with the care of dying children. List some of the factors that have been identified as major influences on caring for the terminally ill child.

REFERENCES

Davies B and Eng B: Factors influencing nursing care of children who are terminally ill: selective review, *Pediatr Nurs* 19:(1):9-13, 1993.

Schonfeld DJ: Talking with children about death, *Pediatr Health Care* 7(6):269-274, 1993.

2. The cure rates for childhood cancer are rising. What are the potential long-term consequences of cancer therapy? Discuss the positive outcomes of cancer treatment in the face of certain negative consequences. How important is the socioeconomic status related to overall adjustment of survivors? Discuss the phenomena of "chronic sorrow" that describes parental psychological reaction to a child who has special health needs.

REFERENCES

Clements DB, Copland LG, Loftus M: Critical times for families with a chronically ill child, *Pediatr Nurs* 16(2):157-161 1889.

Clubb RL: Chronic sorrow: adaptation patterns of parents with chronically ill children, *Pediatr Nurs* 17(5):461-466, 1991.

Hobbie WL and Hollen PJ: Pediatric nurse practitioners specializing with survivors of childhood cancer, *Pediatr Health Care* 7(1):24-30, 1993.

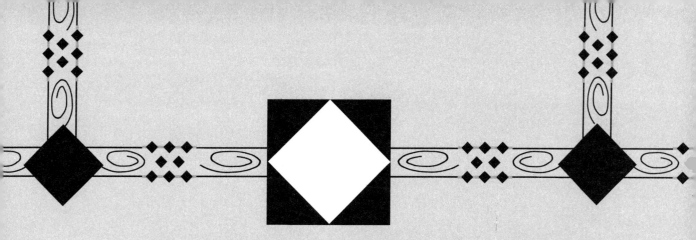

ANSWER KEY
TO
STUDY QUESTIONS
IN
GUIDE BOOK

EXERCISE I   PERSPECTIVES IN MATERNAL AND CHILD HEALTH NURSING

Chapter 1   History and Current Trends in Maternal and Child Health Nursing

1. e, b, f, c, h, a, g, d

2. a. White House Conferences. b. Children's Bureau. c. Social Security Legislation. d. Any four of the following: Program for Children with Special Health Needs (CSHN—formerly Crippled Children's Service); Medicaid (under title XIX of SSA); Early and Periodic Screening Diagnosis and Treatment Program (EPSDT); family planning; foster care; education of public health personnel. e. Project Head Start. f. WIC or Special Supplement Food Program for Women, Infants and Children. g. National Center on Child Abuse. h. Missing Children's Act.

3. a. United Nations Children's Fund (UNICEF). b. World Health Organization.

4. e, d, a, b, c

5. a. 7.3. b. Pulmonary embolism. c. Pregnancy-induced hypertension. d. Hemorrhage. e. Ectopic pregnancy.

6. a. 9.2. b. Lack of access to prenatal care. c. High rate of adolescent pregnancy. d. Low birth weight and disorders related to prematurity. e. Birth defects (congenital anomalies). f. Sudden Infant Death Syndrome (SIDS). g. 5 lb 8 oz. h. 2500 gm. i. Birth before 38 weeks of pregnancy or gestation.

7. a. Increase the span of healthy life for Americans.
   b. Reduce health disparities among Americans.
   c. Achieve access to preventive services for all Americans.

8. b	11. b	14. c
9. d	12. b	15. d
10. a	13. d	

Chapter 2   Contemporary Maternal and Child Health Nursing Practice

1. a. Specialized. b. Health needs. c. Identifiable responses of women. d. Real or potential. e. Childbearing and childrearing. f. Fetus. g. Conception to birth. h. Birth through adolescence.

2. a. Health promotion. b. Prevention.

3. a. Clinical nurse specialist, nurse practitioner, certified nurse midwife. b. Obstetrician, perinatologist, neonatologist.

4. a. Assessment. b. Nursing diagnosis. c. Planning. d. Implementation. e. Evaluation.

5. a. American Nurses Association (Division of MCHN Practice).
   b. Association of Women's Health, Obstetric and Neonatal Nurses (AWHONN—formerly NAACOG).

6. a. Average. b. Education. c. Circumstances.

7. Carefully documenting patient care; obtaining informed consent prior; pursuing continuing education.

8. a. Beneficence (do good). b. Non-malfeasance (do no harm). c. Confidentiality (patient's right to privacy). d. Self-determination (patient's right to decide what happens to his or her own body). e. Justice (allocation of resources).

9. c	11. d	13. d
10. b	12. a	14. c

Chapter 3   The Family in a Multicultural Society

1. "Two or more persons who are joined together by bonds of sharing and emotional closeness and who identify themselves as being part of the family."

2. Bound together by the civil or religious bonds of marriage and adoption.

3. a. Husband, wife, and dependent children living in same household, separate from family of origin. b. Husband and wife alone. c. An adult head of household living with one or more dependent children. d. Nuclear family, nuclear dyad, or single parent family living with one or more dependent parents in the same household. e. Two or more nuclear family households (parents and/or siblings of spouses) living in close proximity and providing mutual support.

4. a. Traditional nuclear. b. 6

5. The single parent.

6. a. Marriage no longer viewed as essential for healthy, satisfying life or childrearing.
   b. Increased acceptance of women employed outside the home.
   c. More tolerance of divorce.
   d. More tolerance of homosexual relationships between consenting adults.

7. a. (1) Affective—meeting emotional needs. (2) Reproductive—ensuring survival of family. (3) Socialization of children; teach children their roles. (4) Health care—health care, food, shelter, clothing, warmth. (5) Economic—securing resources for essential products, services.
   b. The responsibilities of education and religious training have now been largely assumed by schools and churches or other religious organizations.

8. Answers will vary.

9. 2, 3, 1, 5, 4, 6

10. a. *Time*   /orientation to past = values tradition
                                      /orientation to present = now is what is important
                                      /orientation to future = plans for future

    b. *Activity*   /emphasizes doing = values "getting the job done"
                                      /emphasizes being = values self expression; spontaneity
                                      /emphasizes being-becoming = values pursuing personal growth in many areas.

    c. *Interpersonal relationships* /may favor authoritarian; democratic; or individualistic styles of interaction.

    d. *Person-environment*   /may favor positions of mastery; submission; or harmony.
       relationships

    e. *Human nature*   /views mankind as basically evil; good; or neutral.

11. Answers will vary for a and b.
    c. Nurses must be aware of their own cultural values and develop sensitivity toward those of their clients. The ability to recognize when these values differ will enable the nurse to avoid ethnocentric responses and give effective individualized nursing care.

12. d	14. b	16. c
13. c	15. d	17. c

EXERCISE II   HUMAN REPRODUCTION

Chapter 4   Female Reproductive System

1. a. Mons pubis (mons veneris)
   b. Clitoris
   c. Urethral meatus—exit for urine; entrance point for urethral catheter
   d. Vestibule
   e. Vaginal orifice—expansive opening of birth canal
   f. Labium majus
   g. Labium minus
   h. True perineum—may be torn during childbirth; site of midline episiotomy
   i. Anus

2. a. Fimbriated end of fallopian tube
   b. Ovary—female gonad producing ova, estrogen, and progesterone
   c. Fallopian, or uterine, tube or oviduct, middle portion, ampulla—passageway for egg; usual site of fertilization
   d. Fundus or corpus—protects; nourishes developing fetus; helps expel baby
   e. Cervix—neck of uterus; must dilate to make vaginal birth of baby possible
   f. Urinary bladder
   g. Pubic bone
   h. Urethra
   i. Clitoris—center of sexual arousal in female
   j. Labium minus
   k. Labium majus
   l. Pouch of Douglas or cul-de-sac—may be aspirated to detect abnormal pelvic contents
   m. Posterior fornix
   n. Vaginal canal—exit for menses, organ of intercourse, birth canal
   o. Rectum
   p. Anus
   q. True perineum

3. a. Fundus of corpus
   b. Corpus or body
   c. Isthmus
   d. Cervix
   e. Perimetrium
   f. Myometrium
   g. Endometrium

4. a. Sacrum
   b. Pubis
   c. Coccyx
   d. Iliac bones
   e. Iliac crests
   f. Ischial spines
   g. Acetabulums

5. a. Symphysis pubis
   b. Ischial spines
   c. Iliac bones
   d. Coccyx
   e. Sacrum
   f. Sacral promontory
   g. Anterosuperior iliac spines

6. a. Symphysis pubis
   b. Ischial tuberosities
   c. Ischial spines
   d. Iliac bones
   e. Coccyx
   f. Sacrum

7. See text, Figs. 4-10 and 4-11 p. 47.

8. Any four of the following: a. Heredity. b. Infections. c. Poor nutrition. d. Paralysis of one or both extremities. e. Accidents (trauma). f. Poor posture and exercise habits.

9. a. Multiple pregnancies. b. Abnormal fetal positions or presentations. c. Abnormal fetal size or structure (e.g., hydrocephalus).

10. a. External palpation. b. Internal palpation. c. Pelvimetry. d. Ultrasonography.

11. See text, Fig. 4-12, p. 48.

12. See text, Figs. 4-11, p. 47 and 4-15, p. 50.

13. c	16. d	19. c	22. b
14. b	17. a	20. c	
15. c	18. a	21. c	

Chapter 5   Menstrual Cycle

1. A. Pituitary; paired ovaries
   B.

Endocrine gland	Hormone	Action
Pituitary (anterior portion)	Follicle-stimulating hormone (FSH)	Causes follicle and ovum in ovary to mature
	Luteinizing hormone (LH)	Involved in ovulation and beginning the production of progesterone by the newly formed corpus luteum.
Ovaries	Estrogen	Builds up and helps maintain thickened endometrium; initiates and sustains feminine characteristics
	Progesterone	Helps in the deposit of nutritional stores in endometrium in preparation of pregnancy.

2. a. Follicular. b. Luteal. c. Menstrual. d. Proliferative. e. Secretory. f. Ischemic

3. a. First onset of menstruation. b. Excessive (more than 80 ml or longer than seven days) menstruation. c. Bloody vaginal flow between periods. d. Expulsion of egg from follicle of ovary. e. Menstruation. f. Absence of menses due to pregnancy or pathological condition. g. Painful menstruation.

4. Any three of the following: Breast development, widening of hips, fatty deposits in buttocks, pubis, appearance of axillary, pubic hair.

5. See text p. 68 (Fig. 7-1).

6. Any three of the following: a. Counseling. b. Prostaglandin inhibitors. c. diuretics for edema. d. Exercise. e. Well-balanced diet (low sodium and low caffeine intake, vitamin B_6). f. Treatment controversial.

7. d	10. d	13. d
8. b	11. c	14. a
9. c	12. d	15. a

Chapter 6 Male Reproductive System

1. a. Vas deferens, ductus deferens—transport tube for spermatozoa
   b. Pubic bone—covered by mons veneris
   c. Prostate gland
   d. Urethra—passageway for urine or sperm
   e. Prepuce or foreskin—slit or totally or partially removed if circumcision performed.
   f. Glans penis—center of sexual arousal
   g. Urinary bladder
   h. Seminal vesicle
   i. Rectum
   j. Cowper's or bulbourethral gland
   k. Epididymis—coiled tubule where spermatozoa mature
   l. Testis or testicle—producing spermatozoa and testosterone
   m. Scrotum—helps protect testes from trauma; temperature changes

2. a. Maturation of the reproductive system. b. 14.
   c. Any four of the following: enlargement of larynx—deepening of voice; appearance of axillary, pubic, and facial hair; increased musculature; semen production; nocturnal emissions (wet dreams).

3. b	5. b	7. a
4. d	6. c	8. b

Chapter 7 Fertility Management

1. Contraceptive education
   Genetic counseling
   Infertility counseling and methods of fertility enhancement
   Alternative birth technologies
   Adoption

2. The ultimate purpose and potential of the individual and mankind as a whole; how the developmental state of the unborn child affects his or her status as a person or soul; the rights of the unborn versus those of the parents and society; the purposes of the marriage relationship and sexual intercourse; the responsibility and ability of the individual to make and implement decisions involving personal conduct; the role of a deity in the affairs of human beings.

3. a. Fertilization. b. Ovulation. c. Implantation

4. Any five of the following:

Table 7-1 Contraceptive Methods Preventing Fertilization

Contraceptive technique	Advantages	Disadvantages	Failure rate (typical use)	STD/HIV protection
a. Abstinence	No appliances, preparation or expense	At time difficult to maintain—backup method?	0	Yes
b. Coitus interruptus	No appliances, preparation, or expense	Sperm often escape prior to withdrawal	19%	None
c. Periodic abstinence [Natural Family Planning (NFP)]	All forms (1) - (4) No appliance or immediate preparation. Relatively inexpensive. May be acceptable to groups objecting to other forms of contraception	Requires period of abstinence Planning and records necessary	20%	None
(1) Calendar Method rhythm	Simple	Requires period of abstinence Planning necessary	20%	None
(2) Basal Body Temperature	Relatively simple	Required period of abstinence Planning necessary.	20%	None
(3) Changes in cervical mucus "Billings" or "ferning" method	Once learned, relatively simple	Requires period of abstinence More difficult to learn to evaluate More record keeping	20%	None
(4) Symptothermal method employing (1)(2)(3) above and evaluation of libido, spotting, breast tenderness, and cramping, cervical softening, etc.	Women using these methods learn more about their bodies	Requires period of abstinence More complex record keeping	20%	None
d. Periodic use of barrier method during fertile periods identified by using above methods [Fertility Awareness Method (FAM)]	Sexual activity may continue during fertile period but various barriers used	More planning and records necessary	None available	Very limited
e. Male condom	For female, protection responsibility of male Fairly inexpensive Readily available	Must be carefully applied after erection and carefully removed after coitus	12%	Best Protection

Table 7-1 Contraceptive Methods Preventing Fertilization cont'd.

Contraceptive technique	Advantages	Disadvantages	Failure rate (typical use)	STD/HIV protection
f. Female condom	Female able to protect self	Must learn application and removal technique	12%	Best Protection
g. Diaphragm or cervical cap with spermicidal jelly	Fairly inexpensive Highly effective	Must be fitted by physician, carefully positioned by patient. In place no more than 1 hour before intercourse; left in place at least 8 but optimally no more than 24 hours following coitus. Internal appliances, not appealing to some. Diaphragm use associated with bladder infections in some women. Cervical caps should not be used if Papanicolaou smears of cervix are abnormal or if they become abnormal during cap use. Scheduled Pap smears needed.	Diaphragm 18% Cervical cap used by women never pregnant 18% Used by women who have given birth vaginally 36%	Limited
h. Vaginal sponge, containing spermicide nonoxynol-9	Considered highly reliable Sold over the counter One size	An internal appliance, not appealing to some Must be in place no less than 6 hours and no more than 24 hours after coitus	Same as cervical cap	Limited
i. Spermicides—intravaginal cream, foam, jelly, suppository, or tablet	Easy to apply Relatively inexpensive Readily available	Creams, foams, jellies must be applied directly before intercourse and left in place 8 hours. Suppositories and tablets waiting period before coitus necessary—read labels Some users have found them messy, irritating or failing to foam or melt	21%	Limited
j. VCF film	Easy to apply	Must be placed over cervix no less than 5 minutes before intercourse	None available	Limited

5. Any three of the following:

Table 7-2 Contraceptive Methods Preventing Ovulation

Technique	Advantages	Disadvantages	STD/HIV protection
a. The "pill" (combination form)	Use not directly associated with sex act Easy to use Very reliable—failure rate 3% Ability to stop and conceive	Numerous contraindications exist Possible complications including: heart attacks; deep vein thrombosis; hypertension Careful follow-up needed Back-up contraception needed if more than 1 pill missed Questionable use during lactation	None
b. The mini pill (all progestin) Less effective inhibiting ovulation—prevents sperm transport by thickening cervical mucus	All of the above advantages *EXCEPT* less reliable than "combination form" Failure rate 1.1% - 13.2% Does not have negative effect on lactation Less risk of complications associated with combination form	May still have menses or irregular bleeding Watch for profuse or extended flow Back-up contraception needed if pills taken 3 or more hours late Less effective Side effects: same as for a.	None
c. Injectable Progestin—Depo Provera (also thickens cervical mucus)	No internal appliances Not directly associated with sex act Failure rate only 0.3% Injection lasts 3 months	Contraindications: unexplained vaginal bleeding; acute liver disease; breast cancer or blood clots Requires injections Injection lasts 3 months Common side effects: menstrual irregularities and weight gain	None
d. Implants containing Progestin—Norplant (also thickens cervical mucus)	All above advantages EXCEPT duration of effect lasts 5 years Failure rate only 0.09%	Requires subdermal implant with risks of infection, bleeding, and prominent appearance of rod under skin Contraindications and side effects same as for c.	None

6. Any three of the following: a. Vomiting. b. Nausea. c. Irregular vaginal bleeding. d. Breast tenderness. e. Acne. f. Weight gain. g. Possible blood clot formation. h. Hypertensive problems.

7. Any three of the following: a. Heart attack. b. Strokes. c. Deep vein thrombosis. d. Hypertension.

8. See chart "Contraceptive Methods for Preventing Fertilization," 4c through 4d (Answer Key p. 308).

9. a. The state may not intervene with the decision of a woman and her physician to have an abortion during the first 3 months of pregnancy. b. In the second 3 months, before "viability" of the fetus (20 or 24 weeks gestation) the state may regulate the conditions under which abortion is performed but cannot prohibit it. c. After viability the state may prohibit abortion. Most states do so, except to save the life or health of the mother.

10. Webster v. Reproductive Health Services resulted in a Supreme Court decision that would allow individual states to forbid the use of public money to provide abortion services; therefore it may limit access of poor people to abortion services.

11. Female sterilization.
    a. Tubal ligation via *mini-laparotomy* involves abdominal incisions to tie or otherwise occlude the fallopian tubes.
    b. *Band-aid surgery:* Fallopian tubes may be occluded by electrocoagulation, clips or rings following visualization of the operation site through a laparoscope introduced through a small incision at the base of the umbilicus.
    c. *Vaginal tubal sterilization:* peritoneal cavity entered through posterior vaginal fornix with or without a scope similar to laparoscope. Procedure following similar to other laparoscopy technique. Involves increased risk of infection.

    Male sterilization.
    d. *Vas ligation* or *Vasectomy:* usually an outpatient procedure. Twin incisions are made in the area where the scrotum joins the body, just over the vas. The ducts are tied and separated. Portions may be excised. Follow-up sperm counts are made to confirm sterility.

12. Inability to conceive after a year of consistent intercourse without the use of contraception.

13. Any three of the following: a. Microscopic evaluation of semen for number, form, and motility. b. Testicular biopsy. c. Hormone analysis. d. X-ray studies.

14. a. Basal body temperature pattern. b. Determination of LH levels in the urine. c. Biopsy of endometrium. d. Investigation of viscosity of cervical mucus. e. Gas or air studies of patency of oviducts. f. Examination of the uterine cavity and vagina and their secretions.

15. c	17. c	19. b	21. a
16. d	18. c	20. a	22. a

EXERCISE III   PREGNANCY

Chapter 8   Conception and Fetal Development

1. a. Union of male sex cell (sperm) and female sex cell (ovum). b. Fertilized egg. c. Microscopic, solid, mulberrylike mass resulting from early cell division of the zygote. d. Early stage of embryonic growth characterized by a fluid-filled sphere of cells. e. Fingerlike tissue projections of the trophoblast that aid implantation and later as part of developed chorion form the fetal part of placenta. f. Outer layer amniotic sac. g. Inner layer of amniotic sac. h. Small sac that forms RBCs during first six weeks of embryonic development. i. Microscopic primitive beginnings of individual. j. In human beings, the rudimentary structure formed between ten days and two months of intrauterine life. k. Unborn infant after first two months of gestation. l. After-birth; special temporary organ formed partially from chorionic tissue attached to interior wall of uterus, which serves as the intermediary between mother and infant.

2. a. Transfers oxygen and nutrients to the baby. b. Transfers waste products from the baby. c. Manufactures estrogen, progesterone, human chorionic gonadotropin (hCG), and other hormones. d. Provides protection against some substances with high molecular weights. e. Provides possible temporary immunity through transport of maternal antibodies to baby.

3. c, a, d, b, a

4. Fetal function
   g. See answer #2 above
   h. Carries richly oxygenated blood to fetus
   i. Carry poorly oxygenated blood back to placenta
   j. & k. Fetal shunts allowing oxygenated blood to bypass lungs
   l. Brings richly oxygenated blood from the umbilical vein to inferior vena cava

   Destiny following birth of infant
   Expelled, discarded
   Clamped and cut with cord, becomes occluded
   Clamped and cut with cord, becomes occluded
   Normally gradually close after birth
   Ductus arteriosus becomes ligament in days or weeks
   Becomes occluded

5. a. (1) Onset date of last menstrual period
      (2) Fundal height measurement
      (3) Fetal heart detection
      (4) Ultrasound evaluations
   b. Amniotic fluid
   c. (1) Fetal movement identification
      (2) Ultrasound measurements
      (3) Amniocentesis
      (4) Chorionic villi sampling
      (5) Fetal heart monitoring
      (6) Maternal blood analysis
      (7) Meconium stained amniotic fluid
      (8) Fetal blood sampling

6.
a. ??	c. ++	e. +?	g. +?	i. ??
b. ??	d. ++	f. ??	h. +?	j. ++

7. c	11. d	15. a	19. a
8. c	12. b	16. a	20. b
9. a	13. d	17. b	21. d
10. c	14. b	18. c	22. b

Chapter 9   Pregnancy and Prenatal Care

1. a. Capable of life; legally as pertains to infant—a pregnancy of 20 to 24 weeks or more duration, or the delivery of an infant weighing at least 500 g.
    b. A woman who is having or has had one pregnancy.
    c. A woman who has completed one pregnancy of a viable age, or who is carrying her first viable child but is not yet delivered.
    d. A woman who has completed two or more viable pregnancies or who has completed one or more to differentiate her from a first timer.
    e. A woman who has never delivered a viable child.

2. Any four of the following:
    a. Hemodilution generally changes definition of anemia to hemoglobin less than 11 g/dl and hematocrit less than 33%.
    b. Reduction in norms to levels above called physiological anemia of pregnancy.
    c. Leukocyte counts increase. (Average count 5000 to 15,000; with possible unexplained elevations during labor/immediate post partum to 25,000.)
    d. Pulse rate rises 10 to 15 beats/min.
    e. B/P highest when sitting, lowest in left lateral position.
    f. Avoid flat on back positioning to prevent uterine pressure on vena cava resulting in supine hypotensive syndrome.
    g. Blood stasis in lower extremities common, contributing to edema and varicose veins.

3. Any three of the following:
    a. Estrogen causes gums to be more vascular, swollen, may bleed.
    b. Increased progesterone levels related to slowed peristalsis, constipation, heartburn.
    c. Enlarging uterus puts pressure on stomach and colon.
    d. Hemorrhoids may develop due to pressure of uterus and constipation.

4. a. Progesterone causes smooth muscle relaxation of ureters and renal pelvis causing urinary stasis and danger of kidney inflammation.
    b. Uterine pressure on bladder decreases capacity resulting in frequency.

5. a. Ambivalence. b. Sense of well-being. c. Impatience, anxiety.

6. To promote the health and well-being of the pregnant woman, the fetus, the infant, and family up to one year after the infant's birth.

7. a. *Early and continuing risk assessment:* history; physical examination; laboratory tests.
    b. *Health promotion activities:* counseling that promotes and supports healthful behavior; education about pregnancy and parenting; information about the individual's proposed care and treatment.
    c. *Medical and psychological interventions and follow-up.*

8. 90% of all pregnant women will obtain prenatal care within the first 3 months of pregnancy.

9. a. Indications (visible or palpable) of any abnormality or disease involving the external genitalia, vagina, cervix, pelvic cavity, and rectum.
    b. Analysis of diagnostic test results from specimens obtained to identify cervical malignancy or contagious disease.
    c. Evaluation of the size and shape of the bony pelvis.
    d. Detection of the signs of pregnancy.

10. Any six of the following:
    a. Papanicolaou smear (Pap).
    b. Complete blood count
    c. Differential smear
    d. Hemoglobin and/or hematocrit
    e. Screening for sickle cell anemia for unscreened African-Americans
    f. STS or VDRL for detection of syphilis, possible follow-up FTA-ABS
    g. Confirmation of blood type and Rh status
    h. Rubella antibody screen; HI, (HAI) or EIA tests
    i. Hepatitis B (HBsAg) screen; possible immunization
    j. HIV screen should be offered; now is voluntary
    k. Mantoux or Tine skin testing for TB; if positive, chest X-ray
    l. Complete urinalysis and culture or protein and glucose determinations
    m. Identification of disease agent from: vaginal drainage, cervical mucus, blisters (vesicles) by means of microscopic examination. Examples of agents are: *Candida albicans, Trichomonas vaginalis,* Gonorrhea, Chlamydia, Group B streptococcus, Herpes simplex types 1-2.

11. a. Vaginal spotting or bleeding at any time.
    b. Leaking of fluid from the vagina.
    c. Unusual abdominal pain or cramps.
    d. Persistent nausea and vomiting, especially after first trimester.
    e. Marked swelling of the ankles and especially of the hands and face.
    f. Persistent headache or any blurring of vision.
    g. Painful or burning urination.
    h. Foul smelling vaginal discharge.
    i. Chills and fever.

12. Explanations for false answers will vary.
    a. F—visit every four weeks.
    b. F—no hemoglobin or pelvic exam every time
    c. T
    d. F—Rh negative
    e. T
    f. F—gradually increasing movement not sign of jeopardy

13. Yes   G = 5: five pregnancies
         T = 3; three term
         P = 0; zero premature
         A = 1; one abortion
         L = 3; three living children

14. She should be asked to empty her bladder (if still needed, a specimen may be obtained). She will be more comfortable during her pelvic examination and measurements made will be more accurate.

15. (See chart on facing page.)

16. a. Low birth weight. b. Preterm birth. c. Perinatal mortality. d. Hemoglobin.

17. a. 30 mg. b. 12 weeks. c/d. Beef, dark turkey meat, liver, legumes.

18. 25 to 35 pounds.

Nutrient	Role in body/baby building and maintenance	Deficiency (D)/ Excess (E) Problems	Sources
Vitamin B$_6$ Pyridoxine	Amino acid metabolism Protein synthesis	(D) in pregnancy nausea/vomiting, depression Note: long-term use of oral contraceptives may deplete reserves	Animal and vegetable protein and whole grains
Vitamin D	Essential for calcium balance	(E) can cause hypercalcemia; calcification of soft tissues (D) calcium imbalance	Sunlight (synthesized in skin) Vitamin D fortified milk (possible need of supplement 400 IU/day)
Vitamin E	Prevent oxidation of unsaturated fats	(D) cell damage, neurological symptoms	
Folate Folacin (Folic acid)	Necessary for cell division and protein synthesis	(D) megaloblastic anemia; spontaneous AB preterm birth; pregnancy-induced hypertension (PIH); low birth rate; neural tube defects.	Raw fruits, leafy vegetables, liver, yeast, legumes, nuts, whole grains
Calcium	Development of fetal skeleton, teeth Prevent maternal Ca depletion	(D) poor bone and teeth formation; osteoporosis	Milk, milk products, fish (canned with bones), almonds, baked beans, broccoli, tofu, soy beans, figs, dark leafy vegetables, or add nonfat milk solids
Zinc	Cell reproduction and differentiation	(D) fetal growth retardation, congenital malformations, pregnancy-induced hypertension If iron supplement over 30 mg/day, zinc supplementation recommended	Protein foods, milk products
Magnesium	Involved in many biochemical and physiologic processes	(D) can produce tremors, convulsions	Vegetable protein, dark green leafy vegetables, whole grains

19.

Daily Food Analysis for Women

Group	Dietary Analysis 24 Hour Food Intake — Food Consumed – Amount	Servings	NEEDS — Age	Differences	Proposed Diet Modifications to Meet Needs
1 PROTEIN	Animal: Vegetable:		NP 4½ P 6 NP ½ P 1		
2 MILK PRODUCTS			NP — P 3		
3 BREADS CEREALS GRAINS			NP — (4 wg) P 7 (4 wg)		
4 VITAMIN C VEGETABLES FRUITS			NP 1 P 1		
5 VITAMIN A VEGETABLES FRUITS			NP 1 P 1		
6 OTHER VEGETABLES FRUITS			NP 3 P 3		
7 UNSAT FATS			NP 3 P 3		

*NP, nonpregnant; P, pregnant; 4 wg = 4 oz, servings should be whole grain products.
Adapted from Dietary Intake, California Dept. of Health Services MCH/WIC. Nutrition During Pregnancy and the Postpartum Period 5/90.

Sample 24-Hour Dietary Recall (Food Diary): A Pattern to Follow

8 AM	Bran cereal	$1^{1}/2$ cup
	Milk (nonfat)	$^{3}/4$ cup
	Orange juice	6 oz
	Coffee (black)	2 cups
	Water	2 cups
Noon	Sandwich	
	Whole wheat bread	2 slices
	Mayonnaise	1 tsp (approx)
	Lettuce (Romaine)	2 pieces
	Turkey lunch meat	2 slices
	Tomato slices	$^{1}/2$ tomato
	Milk (nonfat)	1 cup
4 PM	Fruit: cantaloupe	1 cup
8 PM	Tossed salad	
	Lettuce	1 cup
	Mushroom (big)	1
	Raisins	$^{1}/8$ cup
	Dressing (oil-based)	1 tbsp
	Spaghetti	
	Spaghetti (noodles)	1 cup
	Spaghetti sauce	$^{1}/2$ cup
	Lean ground beef	$^{1}/2$ oz
	Tomato base—low fat	$^{1}/2$ cup
	Milk (nonfat)	1 cup
	Apple	1 medium size

Daily Food Analysis for Women—A Pattern

Group	Dietary Analysis 24 Hour Food Intake / Food Consumed – Amount		Servings	NEEDS / Age		Differences	Proposed Diet Modifications to Meet Needs
1 PROTEIN	Animal: Turkey lunchmeat	2 sl	1	NP	4½	–3	Add hard boiled egg Increase meat servings
	Lean beef	½ oz	½	P	6	–4½	
	Vegetable:		1½	NP	½	–½	Addition high protein sandwich in afternoon
			0				
			0	P	1	–1	Add nuts, peanut butter-filled celery
2 MILK PRODUCTS	Milk (nonfat)	¾ cup	¾	NP	2	+¾	OK Helps to provide protein ↓ in 1
	Milk (nonfat)	1 cup	1				
	Milk (nonfat)	1 cup	1				
			2¾	P	3	–¼	Add more milk
3 BREADS CEREALS GRAINS	Bran cereal	1½ cup	2	NP	6 (4 wg)	0	OK
	Whole wheat	2 slices	2				
	Spaghetti	1 cup	2				
			6	P	7 (4 wg)	–1	Additional sandwich in 1
4 VITAMIN C VEGETABLES FRUITS	Orange juice	6 oz	1	NP	1	+¾	OK
	Tomato slices	½ tomato	¼				
	Spaghetti sauce (low fat, tomato-based)	½ cup	½				
			1¾	P	1	+¾	OK
5 VITAMIN A VEGETABLES FRUITS	Fruit: Cantaloupe		1	NP	1	0	OK
			1	P	1	0	OK
6 OTHER VEGETABLES FRUITS	Lettuce (Romaine)	½ cup	½	NP	3	+¼	OK
	Lettuce (Romaine)	1 cup	1				
	Mushroom	(1 big)	¼				
	Raisins	⅛ cup	½				
	Apple	med size	1				
			3¼	P	3	+¼	OK even with extra sandwich
7 UNSAT FATS	Mayonnaise	±1 tsp	1	NP	3	–1	OK
	Salad drsg (oil)	1 tbsp	1				
			2	P	3	–1	OK even with extra sandwich

*NP, nonpregnant; P, pregnant; 4 wg = 4 oz, servings should be whole grain products.
Adapted from Dietary Intake, California Dept. of Health Services MCH/WIC. Nutrition During Pregnancy and the Postpartum Period 5/90.

20. a. Enhanced feelings of well–being; quicker return to fitness; help guard physical, emotional and mental health.
    b. Horseback riding; skiing; endurance exercises; contact sports; exercise during high heat, humidity or elevated body temperature.
    c. Pressure on iliac veins and inferior vena cava by the uterus may cause supine hypotensive syndrome: dizziness, sudden decrease in blood pressure.
    d. Drink fluids before and after exercise; limit exercise periods to 30–45 minutes; not exceed their safe attainable heart rate (SHR) or no more than 140 bpm.
    e. Exercises of the pelvic floor involving primarily the pubococcygeal muscle. They may facilitate childbirth, promote healing, aid in restoration of muscle tone; help prevent stress incontinence.

21. a. Prevention can involve eating smaller, more frequent meals of easily digested carbohydrates (every 2–3 hrs); taking fluids other than at meal times; eating dry, high carbohydrate snack before arising; avoiding food odors and getting plenty of fresh air; prescription vitamin B_6 helps some but not all.
    b. Prevention consists of avoiding lying flat after meals, avoiding overeating or highly seasoned fatty or fried foods; having more frequent and leisurely meals. Treatment consists of prescribed antacids such as a mixture of magnesium and aluminum hydroxides, especially before bedtime. Other products high in sodium should not be taken to avoid upsetting electrolyte balance.
    c. Prevention and treatment involves: diet including plenty of roughage, abundant fluids; regular exercise and consistent times for unhurried evacuation. Mild laxatives with health care provider approval.
    d. Prevention and treatment involves: avoiding constrictive bands; crossed legs and long periods of standing. Also resting with legs elevated; wearing well-applied elastic leg wraps or support hose and exercising.
    e. Metronidazole (Flagyl) may be prescribed orally or vaginally and is now the drug of choice for treatment. Sexual partner should be treated also.
    f. For prevention of vaginal infections keeping the perineal area clean and dry and wearing non-tight cotton underpants is helpful. To prevent monilial overgrowth when broad spectrum antibiotics are given for other reasons: oral nystatin (Mycostatin). For treatment, vaginal suppositories and creams of nystatin, miconazole nitrate 2%, or clotrimazole. Intermittent cool tap water compresses to the vulva may help.

22. a. A high level of concentrated cerebral activity can inhibit the reception of other stimuli.
    b. By conditioning the laboring woman to respond neuromuscularly to certain cues and the development of an intense preoccupation that blocks out unwanted stimuli.

23. Any four of the following: Childbirth Education Association, American Red Cross, YMCA, public health departments, adult education departments, medical groups, hospitals.

24. b	27. a	30. d	33. b	36. a
25. b	28. c	31. b	34. c	37. a
26. c	29. a	32. c	35. d	38. b

EXERCISE IV   CHILDBIRTH AND POSTPARTUM

Chapter 10   Mechanics of Labor and Birth

1. a. Size of the bony pelvis (passage). b. Size and position of the fetus (passenger). c. Rhythm and strength of the contractions (powers). d. Mental preparedness of the woman (psyche).

2. a. That part of the baby coming through the pelvic canal first. b. Relationship between a predetermined point of reference on the presenting part of the fetus to the pelvic quadrants of the mother. c. Degree of flexion of the fetal parts, particularly that of the head. d. Relationship of the presenting part to the ischial spines of the pelvis. e. Thinning and shortening of the cervix. f. Enlargement of the cervical canal to a maximum of approximately 10 cm (about 4 inches).

3. a. LOA, b. ROP, c. ROT

4. Any two of the following: a. A posterior position may take longer to rotate and deliver (persistent posterior). b. It may arrest in midrotation. c. The labor may involve more back pain. d. The rotation to OS and delivery may endanger maternal tissues to a greater degree.

5. a. RSP, frank breech. b. LSP, single footling. c. RSP, complete breech.

6.

True Labor	False Labor
Contractions regular. Contractions more frequent. Contractions increase in duration, intensity. Discomfort begins in lower back and radiates to abdomen. Contractions usually intensified by walking. Cervical effacement, dilation are progressive.	Contractions irregular. Frequency usually unchanged. Duration, intensity unchanged. Discomfort primarily in the abdomen. Walking does not affect, or lessen frequency, intensity. Little or no cervical change.

7. a. Descent. b. Flexion. c. Engagement. d. Internal rotation. e. Extension. f. External rotation. g. Expulsion.

8. a. Intensify maternal and infant assessment. b. Use sedation for the mother. c. Stimulate uterine contractions with an oxytocic. d. Prepare for cesarean birth.

9. a. Rise of the uterus to the umbilicus or above. b. Increased firmness and rounded shape of fundus. c. Lengthening of the umbilical cord from vagina. d. Sudden appearance of moderate temporary vaginal bleeding.

10. d	14. c	18. d
11. c	15. d	19. b
12. b	16. d	20. a
13. c	17. a	21. b

Chapter 11   Labor and Birth

1. a. More natural childbirth. b. More control over birth experiences (types of medical intervention). c. More family participation. d. More alternatives in types of care offered. e. Greater access to newborn. f. Lower costs.

2. a. Concern regarding the normal development and health of her infant. b. Fear of a long, drawn-out labor. c. Fear of loss of control. d. Fear of not living up to the expectations of her husband, herself, or hospital staff. e. Concern regarding her ability to cope with the needs of a newborn and a lively $2^1/2$-year-old son. f. Possible financial concerns.

3.

New Name	Traditional Signs	0	1	2
A Appearance	Color	Blue, pale	Body pink, extremities blue	Completely pink
P Pulse	Heart Rate	Absent	Slow (below 100)	Over 100
G Grimace	Reflex response (e.g., to catheter in nostril)	No response	Grimace	Cry, cough, or sneeze
A Activity	Muscle tone	Flaccid	Some flexion of extremities	Actual motion
R Respiratory effort	Respiratory effort	Absent	Slow, irregular	Good crying
			Severely depressed 0 to 3 Moderately depressed 4 to 6 Perfect Score 10	

4. A "burst of energy."

5. a. Lightening and b. engagement approximately 2 weeks before delivery.

6. a. Appearance of show, b. Rupture of bag of waters. c. Regular, increasingly frequent contractions (10-15 minute intervals for 1 hour).

7. See text, pp. 178-180

8. Any three of the following: a. Checking relaxation and timing contractions. b. Giving pelvic support. c. Massage. d. Mouth care. e. Companionship and encouragement. f. Watching for signs of hyperventilation and for the need to change methods of coping.

9. a. Giving complementary support to the couple's efforts. b. Trying not to distract the couple's concentration and relaxation but giving the patient the needed nursing care. c. Trying as much as possible to use the techniques the couple has learned and not to impose her own, if they are different, as long as the couple's techniques are effective and appropriate.

10. See text, p. 166.

11. 120 to 160 beats per minute. Current recommendation is that the observer listen immediately following a contraction or, if possible, during a contraction and the period directly after to detect late deceleration.

12.

Type of deceleration	Problem	Intervention
a. Early deceleration	Possible fetal head compression	No intervention indicated at this time
b. Late deceleration	Possible uteroplacental insufficiency associated with oxytocin use, maternal hypotension, or high-risk pregnancy.	Notify provider. Stop oxytocin administration, turn patient to either side (left preferred), administer O_2, elevate legs (if hypotensive), increase IV. Vaginal exam for fetal scalp stimulation, possible fetal blood pH.
c. Variable deceleration	Possible cord compression	Notify provider Reposition patient, administer O_2, possible vaginal examination to check for prolapsed cord, possible scalp stimulation, fetal blood pH. If moderate, possible amnioinfusion.

13. For a-d, see figures of breathing patterns and 2 methods of bearing down shown for stage II in Table 11-4, pp. 176-177 of text.
    e. (1) Deep breaths usually in through nose and out through mouth; used at beginning and end of contractions to ready body for special breathing, to help relaxation, and to restore normal breathing and gas exchange.
    (2) Point or object somewhere in room used as center of visual concentration.
    (3) Light, patterned abdominal massage usually done with tips of fingers.

14. Midline episiotomy starts at the center of the vaginal rim of the perineum and cuts down vertically. Mediolateral episiotomy begins at same place but angles right or left. See text, p. 189.

15. Answers will vary.

16. a. How long the top of the uterus (fundus) is discerned to be firm or tight as felt by a hand resting lightly on that area.
    b. The peak hardness or firmness of a contraction. It is usually described as mild, moderate, or strong depending on "indentability" of the uterus by the examiner's fingers. Fingers cannot indent the uterus if contraction is strong.
    c. The time from the beginning of one contraction to the beginning of the following contraction.
    d. The time between contractions.
    e. Normally the uterus should be easy to indent.

17. Nursing assessment

18. By letter (rearranged): a, i, h or j, p, c, g, n, k, l, j or h, e, f, b, m, d, o, q.
    By number—outer column: 1, 9, 8 or 10, 16, 3, 7, 14, 11, 12, 10 or 8, 5, 6, 2, 13, 4, 15, 17.

19. b	22. c	25. c	28. b
20. d	23. b	26. a	29. c
21. c	24. b	27. b	30. b

Chapter 12   Pharmacological Pain Management

1. a. A technique or medication that causes memory loss of varying degrees. b. A technique or medication that reduces or eliminates pain. c. A technique or medication that causes sleep. d. A technique or medication that relieves anxiety and quiets the patient. e. A technique or medication that partially or completely eliminates sensation or feeling locally, regionally, or generally. f. A drug that stimulates a cell receptor site and produces a physiological activity. g. A drug that stimulates a cell receptor site and prevents or reverses a specific physiological activity.

2. Fill in Table 12-1

Frequently Used Pharmacological Pain Management Options During Labor and Birth in the United States		
First Stage Labor	**Principal Advantages & Duration**	**Principal Disadvantages**
Types of Systemic Analgesia	**State duration of effective analgesia (Items a, b, c, d)**	

1. Narcotics
 	
    a. meperidine (Demerol)
 	
    b. fentanyl (Sublimaze)
	a. Analgesia effective 2-4 hours
	
	b. Analgesia effective 30-60 minutes
		List 3 special concerns: (Items a, b)
		
		a/b. Maternal/newborn respiratory depression; nausea; itching

2. Agonists/antagonists
 	
    c. butorphonol (Stadol)
 	
    d. nalbuphine (Nubain)
	c. +State 1 special benefit: Analgesia effective without maternal or newborn respiratory depression, 2-4 hours
	
	d. +List 2 benefits: Analgesia effective without respiratory depression. Less incidence of sedation, dysphoria than c.
	Often used to counteract undesirable side effects of spinal or epidural narcotics, 3-6 hours.
		List 3 special concerns (Items c,d)
		
		c/d. May cause sedation, dysphoria, hallucinations. May interfere with subsequent use of spinal or epidural for analgesia effects

Frequently Used Pharmacological Pain Management Options During Labor and Birth in the United States - Cont'd		
First Stage Labor	**Principal Advantages & Duration**	**Principal Disadvantages**
Types of Systemic Analgesia		

3. Tranquilizers (potentiators)
 	
  e. promethazine (Phenergan)
 	
  f. hydroxyzine (Vistaril)
	List 3 benefits and duration: (Items e, f)
	
	e/f. Increase effect of systemic analgesics, decrease narcotic incidence of itching; nausea, 2-6 hrs
		No disadvantages noted in text

Regional analgesia/ anesthesia	**Describe state of mother: (3 aspects)**	**List 6 special concerns or needs**
4. Lumbar epidural block (injection of local anesthetic, e.g., bupivacaine (Marcaine) lidocaine (Xylocaine)	Mother alert, confortable (although sensation of abdominal perineal pressure often noted)	Anesthesiologist, special equipment required. Close nursing observation of: FHTs. P. R. B/P for possible hypotension (danger to unborn infant); urinary retention; numbness; weakness of legs
Second and Third Stages (Vaginal Birth)	**Principal Advantages**	**Principal Disadvantages**
Lumbar epidural block (cont'd)	List 3 benefits: Mother remains alert, confortable Block may be extended to allow for perineal relaxation, episiotomy and repair, or C-section Baby alert	List 2 concerns : Ability to push usually impaired - more forceps used. Delay in ambulation until leg sensation and control present. Indicate 2 rare but serious complications: 1) Injection into dural sac or blood vessel 2) Sensitivity to injected agent

Frequently Used Pharmacological Pain Management Options During Labor and Birth in the United States - Cont'd		
Second and Third Stages (Vaginal Birth)	**Principal Advantages**	**Principal Disadvantages**
5. Subarachnoid (spinal, saddle) block (injection of local anesthetic as above)	List 3 benefits: Mother remains alert, anesthesia effective Baby alert Block may be extended to allow for perineal repair, or C-section	List 6 special concerns/needs: Block usually begun during 2nd stage of labor, a difficult time for mother. Close nursing observation of FHTs, P, R, B/P for hypotension. Possibility of spinal headache < 5% Ability to push usually impaired - more forceps used. Urinary retention. Indicate 1 rare but serious complication: High level anesthesia
6. Epidural and subarachnoid with local anesthetic and *narcotics* e.g., Duramorph and/or fentanyl or sufentanil	Indicate main advantage: All advantages of epidural or spinal. Narcotic injection helps prolong pain control	List 3 side effects of method: Frequent itching; nausea/vomiting from narcotics; urinary retention Indicate 1 rare but serious complication: Delayed respiratory depression. Respiration patterns must be monitored according to protocol in place
7. Pudendal Block	Safety: Safest anesthesia for mother and baby. Main use: Provides anesthesia of perineum for episiotomy	List 2 concerns: Does not relieve contraction pain. Urge to bear down may be diminished, coaching usually compensates.

3. a. Provide childbirth education courses; help her understand and cooperate consciously with what her body is trying to do. b. Maintains a clean, pleasant environment. c. Teach or reinforce techniques of relaxation. d. Help with position changes, application of counter-pressure. e. Continue to encourage. f. Welcome supportive companionship of those she loves.

4. d	7. b	10. a	13. d
5. c	8. d	11. a	
6. b	9. c	12. b	

Chapter 13 Postpartum

1. a. Vital signs—BP,T,P,R, skin color and feel; and pupillary check to detect developing circulatory shock or possible excitement, anxiety, effect of oxytocic infusion or signs of pregnancy-induced hypertension (PIH).
   b. Uterine contractility—consistency, location to detect potential for hemorrhage and filling bladder.
   c. Lochia—type and amount of uterine drainage to detect clots, hemorrhage.
   d. Perineum—appearance, need for ice pack?—prevent swelling, detect hematoma.
   e. Bladder distension—ability to void? Interferes with ability of uterus to contract. I & O evaluation catheterization?
   f. Anesthesia recovery? Ability to feel and move legs? Ambulate?
   g. Pain—affects general well-being, attachment process, ability to move, void?
   h. Hydration and nutrition—evaluate contents, rate and site of infusion—light nourishment provided if tolerated and bleeding not excessive.
   i. Psychological status—provision for reassurance; sharing, rest, and attachment experiences as needed.

2. a. 6 weeks
   b. Involution

3. a. Vital signs; B/P decreasing to low; pulse increasing then becoming slow and thready. b. Pale, clammy skin. c. Apprehension, abnormally dilated pupils, loss of consciousness. d. Uterine contractility—fundus high, soft, or boggy. e. Lochia—profuse, containing clots.

4. At the umbilicus or slightly below.

5. Any 5 of the following: a. Size of baby. b. Multiple births. c.Condition of the uterine muscle, (contracted or relaxed). d. Amount of urine in the bladder. e. Retained placental fragments. f. Uterine infection. g. Number of days following birth.

6. Location of fundus is described according to its position relative to the umbilicus measured up or down by finger widths: at umbilicus: 2 finger widths below = -2, 1 finger width above = +1; and right, left, or midline. Its consistency may be described as firm; firm on massage, boggy—tendency to relax (this condition should be reported). Example of recording: Fundus: firm, midline at umbilicus.

7. a. Uterine massage. b. Increase rate of IV Pitocin—alert staff. c. Putting infant to breast. d. Emptying the bladder.

8. Two hands should be used. One hand is placed at the pubic bone to prevent the relaxed uterus from inverting or prolapsing as the fundus is massaged. If clots are suspected, after the fundus is firm and with the one hand still supporting the lower part of the uterus, the firm fundus is gently grasped by the other hand and pressure is exerted in the direction of the pelvic canal to push out clots already emptied from the uterus into the vagina to the exterior. The nurse should not over-massage. This fatigues the uterine muscle and may lead to more bleeding.

9. Rising fundus often displaced to right or left. b. Puffy area above pubic bone. c. Patient complaints of feeling of fullness—not always reported because of effects of anesthesia. d. Dribbling—voiding of small amount less than 200 ml.

10. If unable to ambulate: a. Measured perineal irrigations. b. Running gurgling water from tap. c. Give pain medication—offer bedpan 20 min. later. d. Have patient blow bubbles through straw or pretend to blow up balloon. If can ambulate, e. Take to toilet. f. Put in shower.

11. a. b

12. a. To prevent infection. b. Eliminate odor. c. Observe the perineum and flow. d. Ease discomfort.

13. Congestion of the breasts, which occurs usually about the third day following birth with increased venous and lymphatic flow and beginning formation of milk.

14. Wear support bras. b. Apply ice packs to breasts. c. Taking analgesics. d. Avoiding breast or nipple stimulation; heat, massage or pumping, breasts. e. Realize it usually resolves in 48 hours.

15. Apply warm wash cloth to breasts or take a hot shower and manually express a small amount of milk to soften breasts before nursing. b. Every 2-3 hr nursing infant but not emptying breasts as this will encourage more milk production not wanted at this time. c. Oxytocin nasal spray to prompt let-down reflex. d. Analgesics (approved by health care provider).

16. Any 10 of the following: a. Observation of dressing/incision. b. Gentle palpation of the fundus but no routine massage. c. Post-anesthetic positioning, turning, coughing, deep-breathing. d. Indwelling catheter care. e. Longer IV care/possible PCA. f. Longer need for pain evaluation/prevention/treatment. g. Abdominal evaluation for distension/gas/peristalsis. h. Longer progressive diet. i. Pericare but no lamp or spray. j. Has less lochial flow. k. Individualized psychological support geared to circumstances/outcome of birth. l. Longer postpartum stay. m. Progressive ambulation.

17. Any 3 of the following: a. Allow freer visiting privileges for family, friends, as the parents desire. b. Provide more access to and communication about sick or abnormal infant. c. Secure pictures of sick or deceased child, lock of hair, footprints, bracelet. d. Realize need for parents to express grief. e. Obtain knowledge regarding mourning process. f. Nurses need to listen and avoid platitudes.

18. a.
19. b.
20. a.
21. c.
22. c.
23. d.
24. b.
25. b.
26. b.
27. c.
28. a.

EXERCISE V   SPECIAL SITUATIONS IN CHILDBEARING

Chapter 14   Complications in Childbearing

1.

(PS) 1.	(PS) 6.
(PS) 2.	(M) 7. g, h, i=(M)(PS)
(PS) 3.	(0) 8. b=(M)(O)
(O) 4.	(PS)(M)(O) 9.
(O) 5.	(O) 10.

2. a. (1) Class III asymptomatic at rest—symptomatic with ordinary activity; Class IV symptomatic at rest and with all activity.
   (2) Near 28 weeks, during labor and in the hours following delivery.
   (3) (Any 5 of the following): pulse >100; respiration >28; dyspnea limiting activity; coughing; rales; chest pain, edema, palpitations, pallor, cyanosis.
   b. (1) Frequency, dysuria, urgency, lower back pain.
   (2) Chills and fever, nausea, vomiting, flank pain (with or without frequency, dysuria, urgency).
   (3) Premature labor and delivery; threat to mother and infant.
   c. (1) Fever, weight loss, fatigue, night sweats.
   (2) Cough, sputum production, hemoptysis, chest pains.
   (3) Treatment during pregnancy; protracted multidrug regimen. Newborn: Prophylactic isoniazid for 3 months.

3. a. Fetal malformations; Spontaneous abortion.
   b. Preterm labor; Premature rupture of membranes; stillbirth.
   c. (1) Chancre.
   (2) Bronze or rose-colored flat or raised scaly rash appearing most significantly on palms and soles of feet; flattened, moist, wartlike lesions on skin or mucous membranes.
   (3) Any 3 of the following: enlargement of lymph nodes, headache, sore throat, aching joints and muscles, spotty loss of hair.
   (4) Possible widespread serious injury to many vital organs such as heart, brain, liver, etc.
   (5) Any 4 of the following: Thick, blood tinged? nasal discharge—snuffles; blistered, peeling hands and feet; fissures around lips and anus; enlarged liver, possible jaundice;
   (6) Sexual intercourse; needles contaminated with infected blood; unprotected contact with lesions (chancre or condylomata lata); transplacental route; unprotected contact with infected infants before sufficient treatment.
   (7) Serology tests; dark-field microscopic studies of secretions.
   (8) Penicillin
   d. (1) Female: Irritating, purulent vaginal discharge, infection of Skene's glands—burning urination. Male: Urethral irritation or discharge.
   (2) Ectopic pregnancy; sterility; generalized infection such as arthritis, abscesses, amniotic infection syndrome; premature delivery, ophthalmia neonatorum—blindness.
   (3) Resistant strains of organism have developed to previously effective medicine.
   e. (1) Most common.
   (2) Both.
   (3) Conjunctivitis or pneumonia.
   f. (1) Herpes simplex virus, type 2, (HSV-2).
   (2) (Any 3 of the following) Fever, dysuria, lymphadenopathy, flulike symptoms.

(3) More painful (severe) and longer in duration.

(4) Irregularly; indefinitely.

(5) 50%; 50%

(6) Cesarean delivery.

g. (1) In fetuses and people immune-suppressed.

(2) Cervical mucus.

(3) Death.

(4) Treatment.

h. (1) Acquired immune deficiency syndrome (AIDS).

(2) Intravenous drug use; sexual exposure secondary to partner's high risk behavior.

(3) Transplacentally; exposure to blood and vaginal secretions; exposure to maternal secretions (e.g., breast milk).

(4) 12 to 15 months.

(5) 2 years of age.

(6) As early in pregnancy as possible;

i. (1) Hepatitis B surface antigen (HBsAg):

(2) Contaminated blood and feces and sexual intercourse.

(3) Infected maternal blood and stool.

(4) Hepatitis B immune globulin (HBIG).

4. a. Hemorrhagic complications: 1st half of pregnancy—abortion, ectopic pregnancy, hydatidiform mole; 2nd half of pregnancy—placenta previa, abruptio placentae, uterine rupture, amniotic fluid embolism and postpartum hemorrhage.

b. Identify 5 or more from the following:

(1) Cautions: never examine bleeding patient vaginally; never give bleeding patient enema; give no food or fluids without order; keep on bedrest.

(2) Observe patient carefully, frequently: level of consciousness, vital signs, FHR, amount and type of bleeding—save evidence if possible, monitor type, duration, interval and relaxation of uterus during contraction pattern. Report uterine tenderness, rigidity.

(3) Communicate findings to staff, physician.

(4) Expect orders for IV fluids, blood analyses, cross-match for transfusion. Check for acceptance of transfusion.

(5) Maintain calm, supportive manner.

(6) Recognize patient's fear for her own and fetus's well being and grief for potential loss.

(7) Provide accurate information regarding condition and ordered treatment.

c. Order: 7, 6, 2, 3, 5, 8, 1, 4, 9

d.

	Abruptio Placentae (Premature Separation of Placenta)	Placenta Previa
Anatomy involved	Placenta is normally implanted high on the uterine wall	Placenta is implanted near or over cervical opening
Possible predisposing factors	Chronic hypertension, local injury, pregnancy-induced hypertension (PIH), rapid changes in intrauterine pressure, fetal weight on the maternal vena cava, dietary deficiency, glomerulonephritis	More common in multiparous pregnancies
Signs and symptoms	(May occur before or during labor) Alteration in contraction pattern, little uterine relaxation, uterus becoming more tender—possibly boardlike. Varying amounts of dark or bright red vaginal bleeding.	Painless, bright red vaginal bleeding in latter part of pregnancy

5. a. (Any 4 of the following) Primipara; pregnancy over 20 weeks duration; edema of the face and hands; sudden 5 lb+ weight gain; low socioeconomic status?; few prenatal clinic visits and poor response to follow-up contacts.
   b. (See facing page)
   c. Underlined: Blood Pressure, Proteinuria, Edema.
   d. Unknown, (Any 4 of the following): Uterine ischemia; superabundant chorionic villi or the first exposure to such tissue; malnutrition; hormonal changes; autoimmune mechanisms; genetic considerations.
   e. (Any 4 of the following): Low economic status; older age; primipara; family history; diabetes; multiple gestation; chronic hypertension; hydatidiform mole; Rh incompatibility.
   f. Convulsion and/or coma.
   g. (Any 8 of the following): Assignment to a quiet room; Check for medical orders for bedrest; Encourage side-lying; Include B/P and FHR with all vital signs every 4 hours; Weigh every AM; Maintain I & O: Inquire regarding daily urine check for proteinuria; Incorporate observations for signs of worsening preeclampsia; Have emergency drug-airway tray, suction, O_2 source and emergency delivery pack easily available; Expect other possible maternal/fetal tests; Watch for signs/symptoms of onset of labor. Psychosocial support essential.
   h. (1) Primarily to prevent or treat convulsions.
   (2) Side effects: vasodilation may cause generalized warmth, diaphoresis; careful dosage necessary to avoid nervous or respiratory system depression. Monitor: Danger signs Resp <14/min; knee jerk absent, urine output <100 ml/4 hrs; fetal distress; magnesium levels should be between 4-10 mg/dl.
   (3) Calcium gluconate (check method, dosage carefully)

SIGNS AND SYMPTOMS OF PREGNANCY-INDUCED HYPERTENSION

Characteristics	Mild Preeclampsia	Severe Preeclampsia
Blood Pressure	>$\frac{140}{90}$ but <$\frac{160}{100}$ or 30 mm systolic ↑ or 15 mm diastolic ↑ following protocol	>$\frac{160}{110}$
Proteinuria (Albuminuria)	300 mg/L/24 hrs or following protocol. 2 separate specimens of 1+,2+	5g or more/24 hrs, or using true clean catch or cath. spec. 3+,4+
Edema	Weight gain of >3 lb or 1.4 kg/wk; >6 lb or 2.7 kg/mo; any sudden weight ↑; output >500 ml+/24 hrs. lower extremity edema	Pronounced edema especially hands and face; accelerated weight gain, output <500 ml/24 hrs.
Neurological Signs and Symptoms	Absent or only occasional headaches; blurred vision, spots before eyes	More persistent headaches and visual blurring, spots. Retinal arteriole spasms on exam.
Other Organ Involvement	None	DTRs, +3+4 clonus, irritability; tinnitus, liver involvement causing epigastric or rt. upper quadrant abd. pain, nausea, vomiting (often: prelude to eclampsia); pulmonary edema; respiratory distress, rales, cyanosis.

6. a. (1)   Rupture of amniotic sac before onset of labor, infant not preterm; major risk maternal infection.
   (2)   Rupture of amniotic sac before term; maternal risk of infection; fetal risk of premature birth and increased morbidity and mortality associated with respiratory distress syndrome (RDS).
   b. (1)   Greater morbidity; mortality for infant; more economic stress on family and/or community resources; greater psychosocial distress for everyone.
   (2)   Tocolytic drugs and/or bed rest and hydration (Additional instruction regarding recognition of signs of labor, fetal well being, and family psychosocial health needed).

7. a. Any infection of the reproductive tract during the puerperium (usually the 6 weeks following birth).
   b. (Any 4 of the following): Time of onset of fever; elevation of fever; other signs or symptoms of infection; culture results.
   c. (Any 5 of the following): Infection of pelvis: abdominal tenderness, pain; foul-smelling lochial drainage; abnormally large uterus; chills; general malaise, anorexia; rise in pulse rate—extension or worsening may cause increased tenderness and distension, nausea and vomiting.

8. a. Pregnancy-induced hypertension; amniotic fluid embolism; thrombophlebitis, abruptio placentae.
   b. Tachypnea; dyspnea; pleuritic chest pain; apprehension; cough.

9. b	14. a	19. c	24. c
10. a	15. a	20. a	25. b
11. a	16. b	21. d	26. c
12. b	17. a	22. a	27. b
13. d	18. c	23. d	28. d

Chapter 15   Special Needs and Age-Related Considerations

1. Developmental level—focused on present, feels invulnerable; Gap between sexual maturity and time of marriage; Pervasive sexual messages in the popular media; Lack of knowledge regarding reproductive function, risk of pregnancy; Social and economic deprivation (perceives few life options): Perception of pregnancy and parenthood as a method to achieve adult status; Family and/or school conflict; Drug and alcohol abuse.

2. Establish a secure sense of identity; Develop meaningful relationships with others; Achieve emotional independence of parents and other adults.

3. a. Rapid growth and development of secondary sex characteristics necessitate changing self-image; Thinking focused on present and herself; Makes initial attempts to be independent of family with peer group.
   b. Physical changes often completed; Still self-centered but problem-solves and thinks about future; testing limits of parental control on personal behavior.
   c. Future oriented, interested in consequences of behavior; Has well-developed sexual identity and better idea of her role in society; Less conflict with family, stable peer relationships.

4. (a) Physical health (b) Psychosocial consequences (c) Premature (d) Low birth weight (e) Adequate prenatal care (f) First (g) Poverty (h) Education.

5. Aid for Dependent Children (AFDC); Medicaid; Food stamps; Payments to health care providers; Housing; Foster care; Day care.

6. Reduce pregnancies among girls aged 17 and younger by 30%; Reduce the proportion of adolescents who have engaged in sexual intercourse to no more than 15% by age 15 and no more than 40% by age 17.

7. (Any 5 of the following) By demonstrating their infants' abilities and reflexes; Teaching them about infant sleep and awake states; Sharing that all parents become frustrated with lack of sleep and infant crying and mentioning methods of relieving that frustration; Teaching that infants do not understand physical punishment; Including involved fathers in this instruction; Recognizing appropriate parenting behaviors; Minimizing do's and don'ts; Reinforcing that parenting is a gradual learning process.

8. Effective birth control methods; Increased number of women pursuing advanced education and careers; Cost of living; Later age for both first and second marriages; An increased number of women in this age group.

9. (Any 5 of the following) Spontaneous abortion; An infant with Down syndrome and other chromosomal abnormalities; Multiple gestation; Gestational diabetes; Pregnancy-induced hypertension; More possibility of chronic maternal disease (renal, diabetic) causing preterm labor; Growth in uterine fibroids may produce preterm labor, lead to malpresentation, difficult labor or postpartum hemorrhage, Placenta previa; Abruptio placentae.

10. (Any 5 of the following) More concerns about the health risk to mother and fetus; Wonder about ability to parent especially if their experience with children is limited or they question their ability to cope with parenthood as they get older; Concerns over changes in relationship to spouse; Changes in lifestyle; Unexpected financial burdens; Troubled about reaction of friends, older potential siblings.

11. d	14. c	17. d
12. b	15. a	18. a
13. d	16. d	19. d

EXERCISE VI   THE NEWBORN

Chapter 16 Newborn Assessment

1. a. 7 lb 8 oz; 3.4 kg. b. 7 lb 0 oz; 3.18 kg. c. 20 inches; 50.8 cm. d. $19^1/2$ inches; 49.5 cm. e. 13 to 14 inches; 33 to 35.5 cm. f. 120 to 160 per min. g. 30 to 60 per min. h. 80-60/45-40. i. 36.5-37° C or 97.7-98.6° F

2. a. Normal greenish-black, sticky, odorless stool of newborn for about 2 days after birth. b. Creamy protective coating on fetus produced by old cutaneous cells mixed with secretion from oil glands. c. Clogged oil glands on face that will clear spontaneously. d. Bluish hands and feet. e. Long hair on body of infant. f. Red marks seen especially at nape of neck, eyebrows, etc., caused by dilation of superficial capillaries or thinness of overlying skin. g. Blue-black colorations seen especially on back of nonwhite newborn; no relation to mental retardation.

3. a. Can see shapes, colors, prefers contrasting colors and faces. Vision improves at 2 mo. b. Should respond to sound at birth. Loud noise produces startle reflex. Infants respond to voices, classical music, bells, chimes. c. Well developed. Identify mother's own breast milk and odor. Have likes; dislikes. d. Taste buds developed at birth. Can taste sweet, bitter, sour, salty. e. Highly developed. Pressure, temperature, pain increasingly felt. f. Rooting; sucking, swallowing; coughing; sneezing; gagging; blinking; grasping; crying? Startle; Moro; plantar; Babinski and tonic neck reflexes.

4. a	7. b	10. c	13. c
5. b	8. d	11. c	14. d
6. c	9. a	12. a	15. b

Chapter 17 Care of the Normal Newborn

1. a. (1) Suctioning excess oral/nasal secretions, (2) Careful supported positioning of infant on side to prevent aspiration.
   b. Any 5 of the following possibilities: (1) Frequent monitoring of infants temperature (4-8 hrs?) (2) preventing excessive heat loss (from drafts, cold surfaces) (3) Use of warm blankets; radiant warmer; some infants need double wrapping; hats. (4) Check infant for signs of developing hypothermia: (e.g., lethargy, apnea, poor feeding, acrocyanosis—after first 12 hours), cool extremities, tachypnea. (5) Recommended air temperature 75-79° F; 24-26° C. (6) Relative humidity 35-50%. (7) Gradual rewarming with preheated radiant warmer if hypothermia develops. (8) Check infant for developing hyperthermia: hot/red skin, sweating (term infants), weak cry, apnea, poor feeding, decreased muscle tone and activity.
   c. (1) Blood glucose analysis for hypoglycemia and observation for signs. (2) Hematocrit level, (3) Signs of abstinence syndrome (withdrawal), toxicology screening.
   d. (1) Referral to parent, wrist/infant ankle and wrist bands. (2) Staff picture identification. (3) No unattended infants.
   e. Any 5 of the following possibilities: (1) Support and protection of head needed. (2) All lifts to have 2 contact points. (3) Neonate not to be lifted by arms. (4) Prone position no longer recommended for healthy newborns during sleep because of study results linking this position to SIDS. (5) Rotation of propped side positions preferred. (6) Not to be left alone flat on back directly after birth because of possibility of aspiration.
   f. (1) IM Vit. K. (2) Monitor cord. (3) Monitor circumcision site. (4) Prevent intracranial bleeding; do not place in head-down positions for prolonged periods.
   g. Any 8 of the following possibilities. (1) Meticulous staff hygiene before starting care. (2) Completed immunizations needed and absence of contagious disease. (3) Hand washing before/after each infant contact. (4) "Clean to dirty" techniques. Use of universal precautions. (5) Frequent diaper changes: H_2O cleansing and drying of perineum. (6) Prophylactic eye medication. (7) Antiseptic cord care and observation. (8) Parental instruction regarding hand washing and infant care. (9) Monitor infant for breaks in skin. (10) Individual infant equipment or disinfection/sterilization techniques used. (11) Health dept. and accreditation standards governing the construction, maintenance and operation of patient care areas.
   h. No answer; see 2.
   i. Any 3 of the following possibilities. (1) Realize the importance of interaction in establishing strong bonds of attachment. (2) Need to recognize cues from infant of readiness to interact (e.g., widening of eye, facial brightening). (3) Need to recognize cues of overstimulation or need for "time out" (turning-away, falling asleep, averting gaze, yawning, etc.) (4) Learning more about infant capabilities and methods of providing appropriate sensory stimulation will help new parents foster innate infant abilities and increase mutual satisfaction. (5) The development of secondary attachments by the infant is helpful in establishing a family support network.
   j. Any 3 of the following: (1) High school, college, or adult education sponsored family education classes. (2) Prenatal-postnatal parent education programs. (3) Well-child visits. (4) Professionally sponsored child care or child development videos. (5) Conversations with "successful parents."

2.

A. Helping the Mother	B. Helping her Infant
1) Helps uterus to contract; complete involution.	1) Curd easier to digest than cow's milk
2) Releases hormone prolactin, producing milk and relaxing effect.	2) Less likely to cause allergies.
3) Promotes mother/infant feelings of attachment.	3) Iron content lower but better absorbed.
4) Delays ovulation and menstruation, but no guarantee of preventing pregnancy.	4) More cholesterol (needed by infant)
5) Lowers risk of breast cancer, osteoporosis?	5) May receive immune factors from mother.
	6) Breast-fed babies have fewer respiratory tract infections.
	7) Breast milk from mother always fresh.

3. a. T; b. T; c. T; d. T; e. F (Use no soap. To avoid trauma and drying, wash usually 1 time/day with clear water.) f. T.

4. a. Iron fortified. b. Infants have developed mild to fatal illnesses because formula has been improperly prepared. c. Room. d. 45° angle. e. Full of milk. f. (1) Cause pain. (2) Decrease appetite. (3) Promote regurgitation. g. Equipment/Supplies (capped formula bottle, nipple, bottle brush, soap or detergent, saucepan, can opener, spoon). Formula as prescribed: ready to use, liquid concentrate, powder. STEPS: 1. Use a formula bottle that has been washed in the dishwasher or in warm, sudsy water, rinsed in hot water, and air dried. 2. Use a nipple that has been carefully washed and rinsed. Make sure that the nipple holes are open. Some references also recommend boiling the clean nipple 3 to 5 minutes. 3. Shake the formula can well (if liquid type); wipe off the lid before opening. (4) Measure the ingredients needed for one feeding into the bottle. Read the directions carefully. Be sure that you understand what dilution (if any) is to be made. (5) Add warm tap water to the bottle in the amount the directions indicate. Boil bottled water or well water for 5 minutes (neither contain chlorine and can become contaminated). (6) Mix with a clean spoon. (7) Unless you are planning to refrigerate the formula, feed immediately; do not save partially consumed bottles of formula from one feeding to the next or for more than an hour. (8) Prepared formula may be stored in the refrigerator for 48 hours. (9) Bring refrigerated formula to room temperature by placing the bottle in a warm pan of water. Do not microwave—hot spots can result.

5. a. Observing behavior—does the infant seem content, or is the infant a short sleeper and irritable? Infant should have vigorous activity and be generally happy.
    b. Watching for signs of dehydration from poor fluid intake: (1) Fewer than 6 to 8 wet diapers per day. (2) Dark, concentrated urine; dry, hard stools. (3) Dry mucous membranes. (4) Dry skin with little elasticity (poor turgor). (5) Low-grade fever (Note that the most common cause of low-grade fever is dehydration, although the nurse shouldn't overlook the possibility of infection). (6) Elevated specific gravity (above 1.020). (7) In severe cases, sunken fontanels.
    c. Measuring intake; (1) This is routine with bottle-fed babies. (2) If the infant is ill, measuring may be ordered for breast-fed babies. They are weighed directly before and after feeding without a blanket or clothes change (1 g = 1 ml; 30 ml = 1 oz). (3) Intake should be evaluated in terms of a 24-hour period and not individual feedings.
    d. Measuring weight gain: (2) All babies lose weight directly after birth, which should cause no concern unless the weight loss approaches 10% of the birth weight. Bottle-fed babies regain their birth weight more rapidly than most breast-fed babies. (2) After weight gain is reestablished, a gain of about 1 ounce a day is average, equaling about 6 ounces a week. At the end of 5 months most babies double birth weight.

6. d	10. a	14. b	18. a
7. a	11. c	15. b	19. c
8. b	12. c	16. d	20. d
9. d	13. a	17. d	

Chapter 18 The Newborn with Special Needs

1. a. An infant born before the end of the thirty-seventh week of gestation regardless of weight (using menstrual age).
    b. Infant born between the beginning of the thirty-eighth week and the end of the forty-second week of gestation regardless of weight.
    c. Infant born after 42 weeks' gestation regardless of weight.
    d. Infant whose birth weight falls below the tenth percentile on the growth curve.
    e. Infant weighing less than 2500 gm or $5\frac{1}{2}$ lb at birth.
    f. Infant whose weight is less than 1500 grams.

2. a. Low socioeconomic status. b. Teenage pregnancy. c. Multiple birth. d. Excessive smoking. e. Lack of prenatal care.

3.

Characteristic	Normal Newborn	Premature
Subcutaneous fat	More fat, less wrinkled	Less fat, more wrinkled
Lanugo	Less	More
Breasts	7-10 mm breast tissue	Less than 7 mm breast tissue
Normal sole creases	Developed	Absent or poorly developed
Ears	Stand out, incurving to lobe	Limited incurving, very soft
Scarf sign	Absent	Present
Tendon of Achilles	Lengthened	Shortened
Ability to regulate body temperature	Fairly limited	Very limited
Susceptibility to infection	In jeopardy	In great jeopardy
Iron reserves	Normal for age	Insufficient

Also refer to chart on p. 337 of text.

4. Any six of the following: a. Bulging fontanel. b. Abnormal increase in head size. c. Vomiting. d. Unequally dilated pupils. e. Unreactive or abnormally dilated pupils. f. Irritability. g. Lethargy. h. Irregular respiration. i. Slow pulse. j. High shrill cry. K. Twitching. l. Sunset sign.

5. Ventriculoperitoneal shunts are the most common. Also used are lumboperitoneal and ventriculoatrial shunts. b. (1) An occluded shunt no matter what the cause and (2) an infected shunt.

6. Any five of the following: a. Large tongue. b. Slanted eyes, c. Short hands and fingers. d. Little finger bent in. e. Deep horizontal crease on palm. f. Large space between great and small toes. g. Decreased muscle tone. h. Increased joint mobility. i. Short length. j. Small head flattened from front to back. k. Typical dots on iris. l. Low birth weight. m. Lethargic.

7. Translocation type of Down syndrome.

8. 1 in 650 live births. Mothers bearing children after 40 years of age, near the end of their reproductive period, are at greatest risk.

9. Any three of the following: a. Galactosemia. b. Phenylketonuria. c. Congenital hypothyroidism. d. Birth injury. e. Intrauterine infection.

10. a. Mother must be Rh negative (Rh–) for D and D^u; child must be Rh positive (Rh+) for D; child's red blood cells must pass through placenta and enter mother's circulation, and mother must build up antibodies; antibodies must then return to the fetal bloodstream for complications to occur.
    b. If an Rh– woman has an Rh– mate or if Rh immune globulin (RhoGAM or equivalent) is given to an unsensitized woman within 72 hours after delivery of the Rh+ fetus or abortus. (Some physicians are also giving the immunization at 28 weeks' gestation to protect against the consequences of unknown antepartal bleeding, as well as following amniocentesis).

c. Any four of the following: (1) Early jaundice. (2) Lethargy. (3) Poor sucking. (4) Twitching. (5) Spasticity. (6) Bilirubin titer elevated. (7) Anemia. (8) Immature RBCs seen in laboratory tests.

d. Fluorescent lamp therapy; exchange transfusion.

e. Intrauterine transfusion.

11. a, e, c, f, b, d.

12. The lumbar spine is divided and a portion of the posterior wall of the spine is missing. The meninges protrude through the spinal opening and nerve tissues are found in the herniated sac.

13. a. Fecal and urinary incontinence. b. Lower extremity paralysis or weakness. c. Lower extremity loss of sensation. d. Developing hydrocephalus.

14. To reduce the possibility of infection.

15. a. Clubfeet. b. Dislocated hip.

16. Usually between 6 and 10 weeks because a cleft lip may create special feeding problems.

17. a. Elbow restraints to keep baby off of abdomen to prevent trauma to suture line. b. To reduce sucking movements, nothing is placed in the mouth unless specifically ordered. c. Try to keep from crying. d. Use of an infant seat to avoid trauma to the suture line.

18. Orders to keep suture line clean with water, saline, or hydrogen peroxide, application of antibiotic ointment.

19. b	21. b	23. c	25. c
20. c	22. d	24. d	26. d

Chapter 19   Intensive Care of the Newborn

1. The earliest and maximum degree of medical and nursing care for the infant.

2. The neonatal transport team usually consists of: a pediatrician, neonatal nurse clinician or practitioner, a respiratory therapist, and one NICU staff nurse.

3. Any six of the following. a. No prenatal care. b. Poor nutrition. c. Poor obstetrical histories. d. Pregnancies involve coincidental medical illnesses. e. Abnormal presentation or fetal size. f. Multiple births. g. Premature rupture of the membranes. h. Inappropriate maternal anesthesia or analgesia. (See text, p. 364)

4. The range at which his normal body temperature can be maintained with least expenditure of energy.

5. The knowledgeable, alert nurse.

6. More

7. He has good sucking and swallowing reflexes.

8. Any five of the following: a. Respiratory distress (rapid respirations, grunting, apnea). b. Poor feeding. c. Vomiting. d. Temperature instability. e. Jaundice. f. Lethargy.

9. Any two of the following: a. Are overweight. b. Have immature lungs and RDS. c. Are hypoglycemic.

10. Any three of the following: a. Dry skin, some peeling. b. Long fingernails. c. Alert appearance. d. Susceptible to hypoglycemia. e. Meconium staining of the skin.

11. Ideally he would be able to see his daughter right away. a. He should be told the visiting policies and telephone number of the NICU. b. He should be taught how to wash and gown. c. He should be taken to her and encouraged to gently touch his daughter. d. Any procedures and equipment being used should be explained.

12. Any four of the following: a. Increasing respiratory rate (over 45 breaths per min at rest). b. Nasal flaring. c. Increasing retractions. d. Grunting respirations. e. Cyanosis in room air. f. Typical x-ray film. g. Decreasing arterial Po_2 (less than 70) and increasing Pco_2 (more than 45). h. Increasing acidosis.

13. Wendy is unable to get sufficient air in her lungs because of the increased effort she must exert to open her collapsed air sacs with each breath. CPAP is one method of preventing complete alveolar collapse and maintaining proper oxygenation in treatment of the baby. An endotracheal tube is placed in the baby's throat to help her get the best possible oxygen exchange. CPAP apparatus is attached to the tube. As the infant's lungs mature, the amount of CPAP and oxygen concentration are gradually decreased.

14. She is being maintained on assisted ventilation, which predisposes her to infection.

15. Any two of the following: a. Emboli. b. Hemorrhage. c. Sepsis.

16. a	18. a	20. b	22. d
17. a	19. b	21. d	23. d

EXERCISE VII   DEVELOPMENTAL HEALTH PROMOTION

Chapter 20   Genetic and Environmental Factors

1. a. Increase in structure. b. Increase in function. c. Process whereby inherited tendencies begin to unfold, independent of any special practice or training. d. Elements of inheritance, defined lengths of deoxyribonucleic acid (DNA) on structures called chromosomes found in every cell's nucleus. e. The construction of a chart that uses standard symbols to designate family members, their relationships, and other pertinent information. f. Microscopic structures within the nucleus of a cell that contain a species' genes.

2. a. Certain types of mental retardation (e.g., Down syndrome, arrested hydrocephalus, some forms of cerebral palsy).
   b. (1) End stage renal disease, (2) Chronic heart disease, (3) Uncontrolled insulin-dependent diabetes type I, (4) Malabsorption syndromes (e.g., celiac disease, cystic fibrosis).

3. They occur in an orderly sequence. b. Although continuous, they are characterized by spurts and periods of relative rest. c. They progress at highly individualized rates from child to child. d. They involve specific structures that mature at different ages. e. They represent a total process involving the whole child.

4. Every child is different. No two children grow at the same rate. Each child has his own unique growth timetable.

5. a. Genetic (Inhibit growth): Cystic fibrosis, sickle cell disease. (Enhance growth): Early detection and treatment of phenylketonuria.
   b. Environmental (Inhibit growth): Poor nutrition, child abuse. (Enhance growth): Good nutrition, happy home life.

6. a. DNA. b. Chromosomes, c. 46. d. Half, or 23. e. Half, or 23. f. Autosomes. g. Karyotype. h. Various failures in the production of ova and sperm within the two gonads (meiosis). i. Abnormal segregation of chromosomes during the first several mitotic divisions of body cells (mitosis).

7. a. 50%

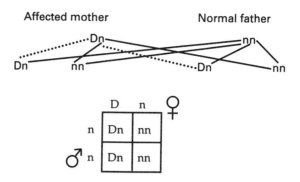

b. Heterozygous
c. Achondroplasia (a form of dwarfism); Huntington's chorea

8. a. 25%

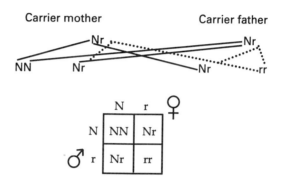

b. Homozygous
c. Any two of the following: (1) Phenylketonuria. (2) Sickle cell disease. (3) Albinism. (4) Tay-Sachs disease.

9. a. X-linked recessive inheritance involves genes located on the X chromosome. The female is the carrier because fathers give male offspring only a Y chromosome. Each male child of a female carrier has a 50% chance of being affected, and each female offspring has a 50% change of being a carrier. b. Any two of the following: (1) Hemophilia. (2) Duchenne's muscular dystrophy. (3) Hurler's syndrome.

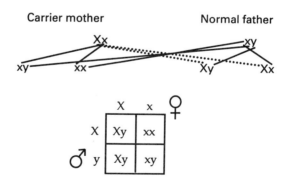

10. The purpose of the US Genome Project is to create a complete map and sequence of all 3 billion base pairs of DNA that make up the human genetic complement.

11. The ultimate goal of the Human Genome Project is to provide information to help understand genetic disease in general.

12. Usually at 16 weeks but can be done between weeks 10 and 14.

13. Yes. Another technique, chorionic villi sampling, provides an alternative approach for prenatal diagnosis.

14. Nutrition

15. a. No. b. Tetracycline antibiotics taken by his mother during the prenatal period or taken by John before age 8 years.

16.

	Stage	Sample behavior
a.	20 weeks	Looks and approaches
b.	24 weeks	Looks and crudely grasps with whole hand
c.	36 weeks	Looks and deftly grasps with fingers
d.	52 weeks	Looks, grasps with forefinger and thumb, deftly releases
e.	15 months	Looks, grasps and releases to build a tower of blocks

17.

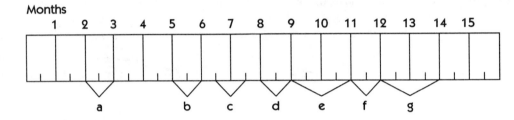

18. Approximately 10% of children scored higher than both of Jane's sisters and approximately 90% of children scored below Jane's sisters in height and weight.

19. Jane is between the tenth and twenty-fifth percentiles for height and at the tenth percentile for weight.

20. Jane can best be evaluated by comparing her height and weight from time to time with her past statistics. You can encourage the mother to have Jane's height and weight checked again in about 6 months and say that no conclusion can be made at this time.

21. d		26. c		31. a.		36. d
22. a		27. c		32. a		37. a
23. d		28. a		33. a		38. a
24. c		29. a		34. b		39. b
25. d		30. b		35. d		40. d

Chapter 21   Developmental Assessment

1. a. 5-7 oz. b. 5 months. c. 1 year. d. 10 inches. e. 3 to 5 inches. f. 10 to 14 years (girls) and 12 to 16 years (boys). g. 7 to 9 months. h. 5 to 7 months; lower front (central incisor). i. 24. j. 3.

2. To detect developmental delays in young children.

3. b		7. c		11. c		15. c
4. b		8. d		12. c		16. c
5. c		9. a		13. d		17. c
6. b		10. c		14. c		

Chapter 22   Child Health Promotion

1. a. (1) Promote health. (2) Prevent disease. (3) Provide anticipatory guidance for developmental and parenting issues. (4) Offer appropriate counseling about child rearing practices and commonly encountered child behavior patterns. (5) Keep records of the child's individual health history and his personal height, weight, and BP plotted in graph form.
    b. The infant is usually scheduled to visit the nurse practitioner or physician within 1 week after birth and then once per month during the first 6 months and every 2 months until age 1 year; during the second year 2 visits or as necessary, and thereafter once per year or as necessary.
    c. Before any apparent problems, and prior to 3 years of age.

2. a. (1) Provide heat and energy. (2) Build and repair tissues of the body. (3) Regulate body processes.
    b. (1) Oxygen. (2) Water. (3) Carbohydrates. (4) Proteins. (5) Fats. (6) Minerals. (7) Vitamins. (8) Fiber.

3. 100 ml/100 kcal. The infant must receive equal fluid intake to account for normal fluid losses.

4. The end products of protein digestion are amino acids. Complete proteins are essential for growth and development. They must all be present at the same time in the bloodstream to form normal tissue and function properly.

5. Complete proteins contain all the essential amino acids. Examples of complete proteins are milk, meat, eggs, cheese, and fish. Incomplete proteins do not contain all the essential amino acids; they are found in vegetables and grains.

6. a. Vitamin A. b. Vitamin D.

7. a. Vitamin A. b. Vitamin D. c. Vitamin E. d. Vitamin K.

8. a. Iron. b. Calcium.

9. The amount of heat needed to raise the temperature of 1 liter of water 1° C.

10. a. 4. b. 4. c. 9.

11. By the fourth month.

12. a. Self-feeding skills develop in the second 6 months of life. At 7 months an infant can hold own bottle. At 8 months an infant can feed himself or herself a cracker. b. Self-feeding is usually accomplished between 12 and 18 months.

13. a. Hepatitis B is given to the newborn before discharge.
    b. (1) Diphtheria, (2) Tetanus, (3) Pertussis, (4) Polio, (5) Measles, (6) Mumps, (7) Rubella, (8) Hepatitis B.
    c. Advisory Committee on Immunization Practices (ACIP) and the American Academy of Pediatrics (AAP).
    d. (1) Moderate or severe illness. (2) During administration of steroids, irradiation, and anticancer drug therapy. (3) Live attenuated vaccines against measles, rubella, and mumps are not given during pregnancy, in cases of generalized malignancy, or if immune globulin, plasma, or blood has recently been administered.
    e. 4 to 6 months.
    f. Passive immunized (administration of antibodies produced by other humans or animals) may confer temporary protection against a few diseases. Active immunity (formation of antibodies by the patient himself) confers long-lasting immunity against disease.

14. a. Age of child (young child most vulnerable). b. Sex of child (males more vulnerable at all ages). c. Nonwhite child has higher incidence of injuries. d. Most injuries occur during spring and summer months. e. High percentage of injuries occur in the home.

15. a. It is an "age of curiosity," and young children explore the environment in many different ways, one way being tasting.
   b. Any five of the following: (1) Keep all drugs and poisonous substances and household chemicals locked and out of reach. (2) Do not transfer or store poisons or inflammable materials in food containers or bottles. (3) Never tell children that flavored medicine is candy. (4) Discard old medicines down the drain before throwing away the container. (5) Always read the label before giving medicine. (6) Always return medicine to its proper place.
   c. (1) If child has ingested corrosives, lye or strong acids, strychnine, or hydrocarbons (such as kerosene, gasoline, fuel oil, paint thinner, and cleaning fluid). (2) If child is unconscious. (3) If child is convulsing.
   d. Toddlers are most likely to ingest poisons, and syrup of ipecac is an emetic drug. Dose; 15 ml for children over 1 year followed by 1 cup of water; repeat no more than once, if necessary, in 15 to 30 minutes.

16. d	23. b	30. d	37. b
17. d	24. b	31. d	38. b
18. b	25. b	32. a	39. c
19. b	26. b	33. b	40. c
20. b	27. b	34. b	
21. c	28. c	35. a	
22. c	29. c	36. b	

Chapter 23   Laboratory Screening in Child Health

1. Explain procedure to child: help support or restrain child.

2. a.

Blood	Newborn—higher than adult Child—4.5 to 6/mm^3
WBC	At birth—averages 20,000/mm^3. By 3 years—4500 to 11,000/mm^3.
Hematocrit	Newborn—45% to 60% 2 to 6 months—35% +
Hemoglobin	Newborn—14.5 to 22.5 g/dl 2 months—9 to 14 g/dl

   b.

Urine

Color	Depends on hydration/medication
Acetone	Negative
Albumin	Common in newborn; negative in child
Glucose	Negative
Cells	Few epithelial, few WBC
Casts	Rare hyaline seen
Specific gravity	1.002 to 1.010 in newborns, 1.003 to 1.030
pH	4.5 to 7.5 (usually acid)

3. Answers probably include the following information: Cathartics and cleansing enema might be ordered on the previous day or morning of the test. A clear liquid diet may be given 1 day before the test until it is completed. A barium enema is given in the x-ray department when the patient is under the fluoroscope; the examination takes 1 to 2 hours. An enema or a cathartic might be ordered after x-ray films are completed to remove contrast media.

4. The night before the test the patient may have a light supper; no foods, fluid, or medications are given after midnight until 6-hour x-ray studies are completed; the x-ray department gives barium under the fluoro-scope. The patient is given nothing by mouth until the x-ray department releases him after the 6-hour follow-up study. If 24-hour studies are ordered, no enema or cathartic is given until the studies are completed; check for enema or cathartic orders when the test is completed.

5. d, c, a, b, e.

6. d	9. c	12. c	15. a
7. a	10. d	13. d	
8. c	11. d	14. a	

EXERCISE VIII THE HOSPITALIZED CHILD AND FAMILY

Chapter 24 The Hospitalized Child

1. Any three of the following: a. Developmental level. b. Previous experience. c. Coping strategies. d. Seriousness of the diagnosis. e. Available support systems.

2. Separation anxiety occurs when parents are unable to come to the hospital for prolonged periods and when the child is exposed to numerous traumatic factors, resulting in frustration of those inborn needs that are normally met in a family environment. Separation anxiety is characteristic of all young children who have established a healthy parent-child relationship and is most likely to effect children under age 4.

3. a. Protest: child cries aloud. b. Despair: child becomes apathetic and withdrawn. c. Detachment: child begins to show more interest in surroundings and is more responsive to nursing attention.

4. After the child returns home

5. Explain to Mrs. Green why Tim is crying. Tell her that all children who have established a healthy mother-child relationship cry when their mothers leave and sometimes cry when their mother returns. Encourage Mrs. Green to tell Tim in words that he can understand when she will come back.

6. a. Colorful booklets and pamphlets. b. Telephone calls. c. Hospital tours. d. Preadmission orientation parties. e. Movies. f. Puppet show. g. Teaching dolls. h. Educational television.

7. c	12. d	17. c	22. c
8. d	13. a	18. a	23. d
9. a.	14. c	19. c	24. d
10. a	15. a	20. a	25. a
11. c	16. b	21. c	26. c

Chapter 25   Hospital Admission and Discharge

1. To determine dosages of medications and general condition and progress

2. Diarrhea and/or vomiting, problems regarding intake and/or output. Weights are checked routinely in the morning before breakfast.

3. A child who has a seizure disorder or poor muscle control; one who has difficulty keeping his mouth closed, or has had oral surgery, or breathing difficulties. (Axillary temperatures are recommended for children under age 6.)

4. a. 100° F (37.8° C). b. 100.4° F (38° C).

5. Rectal temperatures are now generally not recommended for children under 6 years and are contraindicated for young infants, persons with cancer, diarrhea, or rectal pathology.

6. It is too difficult to secure an accurate radial pulse rate.

7. Place the stethoscope between the left nipple and the sternum. In most cases, time for 30 seconds and multiply by two for the very young child.

8.
Approximate pulse and respiration rates

Age	Pulse	Respiration
Birth	110-150	30-50
1 month to 1 year	100-140	26-34
4 years	90-110	20-30
6 to 10 years	80-100	18-26
12 years	76-90	16-24

9. The cuff bladder should be 20% wider than the diameter of the extremity or should cover two thirds of the upper arm (from the shoulder to the elbow).

10.

Problem Area	Observation
Growth and development	Age and sex; special physical considerations, such as orthopedic problems, nutritional status, cosmetic defects, prostheses, and surgically created stomas, history of seizures and general health, cultural, intellectual and emotional considerations.
Skin manifestations	Any unusual color, birthmarks, bruises, rashes, or scars; body or head lice; personal hygiene.
Neurologic system manifestations	Level of consciousness; equality of pupils; bulging fontanel; paralysis or weakness; tremors/twitching.
Other important signs/symptoms	Diarrhea, nausea/vomiting, abdominal distention, nasal drainage, coughing, difficulty voiding, weak stream.

11. Any five of the following: a. Preplanning and needed teaching. b. Arrangements for transportation. b. dismissal in AM. c. Write specific instructions regarding medications/procedures. e. Follow-up appointments.

12. b	15. d	18. a	21. d
13. d	16. a	19. b	
14. b	17. b	20. c	

Chapter 26   Health Maintenance of the Hospitalized Child

1. Failure to check the diet can upset treatment and threaten the health of the patient. a. Developmentally appropriate, b. Compatible with the diet order, c. Cultural preferences, d. Religious background, and e. Any allergies.

2. a. Allergic children. b. Those failing to thrive. c. Those with diabetes or other metabolic problems.

3. Does she drink from a cup, glass, or bottle? Can her mother come in to feed her? What kinds of fluids does she drink at home?

4. 7.35 to 7.45.

5. a. Lungs, b. Kidneys, c. Buffer systems.

6. Any four of the following: a. Apathy. b. Deep rapid breathing (Kussmaul's respiration). c. Disorientation. d. Weakness. e. Coma.

7. Any four of the following: a. Diabetes mellitus. b. Starvation. c. Kidney insufficiency. d. Severe diarrhea. e. Salicylate intoxication. f. Excessive parenteral sodium chloride.

8. Fluid intake must equal fluid output.

9. To maintain plasma volume, which is decreased as a result of diarrhea, interstitial fluid shifts into plasma, causing dehydration manifested by loss of turgor and wrinkled skin.

10. Any four of the following: a. Grayish skin. b. Rapid and weak pulse. c. Elevated temperature. d. Low BP. e. Scanty urinary output. f. Apathy. g. Possible seizures.

11. a. He ingests and excretes a relatively greater daily water volume, b. The infant's body surface in relation to his body weight is three times that of the older child. Therefore he loses a relatively greater amount of fluid through the skin and gastrointestinal tract. c. His high metabolic rate produces more waste products that must be diluted for excretion. d. His immature kidneys are less able to concentrate urine, adding to the volume of urine. e. Accumulation of acidic wastes stimulates respirations, causing greater evaporation through the lungs. f. He may react to infections with higher temperatures associated with greater water loss.

12. a. Kidneys. b. Lungs, c. Skin. d. Intestines.

13. d, e, b, f, c, a.

14. Physically—develops new abilities. b. Intellectually—acquires knowledge about himself. c. Emotionally—uses play to express what he is thinking and feeling. d. Socially—learns to relate to and interact with others.

15. a. Developmental age. b. Safety. c. Durability.

16. Play is a learning activity that is vital to growth.

17. Answers will vary. The following are suggestions:

Age	Interest	Toys	Books
Infant	Toys that attract eyes or make little sounds; toys that he can grasp but now swallow	Bright hanging mobile, bells, rubber toys that squeak or ring	"Pat the Bunny," Dr. Seuss books
Toddler	Toys that enable parallel play, provide security, help develop large muscle coordination	Nest of blocks, trucks and cars, cuddly toy animals or dolls, mallet and pegs	Large linen picture books, nursery rhymes, ABC books, farm and zoo animal books
Preschool	Toys that stimulate imagination, develop creative abilities	Nurse-doctor kit, trains and tracks, action figures, crayons and color books simple puzzles, clay	Dr. Seuss books, Golden Books, once-upon-a-time stories
Early school age	Application of mental as well as physical skills, playing with children of same sex	Craft sets, models, painting, spool knitting, bead work	Comic books, riddle books, crossword puzzles, fairy stories.
Preadolescent	Group activities	Card games, checkers, picture viewer	Comic books, biographies, adventure stories.

18. Placing a medication in a baby's formula is precarious. Gena might not take all the formula, and it would then be difficult to estimate how much of the medicine she took.

19. Place medicine in an empty nipple, and let Gena suck on it; she can try a small medicine cup, rubber-tipped medicine dropper, or syringe. Medicine should be given to the child in a sitting position if possible.

20. Syringe, rubber-tipped medicine dropper, or nipple.

21. 22-gauge, 1-inch.

22. Lateral or anterior thigh, deltoid muscle, or soft tissue inferior to iliac crests.

23. It is not well developed, and it is possible to damage the sciatic nerve.

24. Gentle suction; for example, use a bulb syringe.

25. The child should be lying down with his head tilted back over a folded towel or small pillow. The dropper should be pointed slightly toward the top of the nasal cavity. The child should remain in that position for several minutes after the medicine is given.

26. Find out what he likes; offer Paul a choice, if possible; sit down with him and talk to him while he drinks.

27. Fluids allowed: Popsicles or ice cubes, Jell-O, water, milk, soup, ice cream, and juice—dependent on Paul's allergies.

28. Thirty drops per minute.

29. a. The intravenous site should be checked frequently for inflammation or infiltration. b. Observe the rate of flow. c. Child's response to fluid therapy must be observed. d. Child must be appropriately restrained.

30. Conventional intravenous fluid therapy cannot sustain life. total parenteral hyperalimentation provides glucose, proteins, lipids, minerals, vitamins, and fluid necessary for normal growth and weight gain.

31. By use of a large vein the feeding can be rapidly diluted, and there is less risk of thrombosis and phlebitis.

32. Yes, but risk of tissue damage is considerably greater than when the jugular vein is used.

33. a. Glucose. b. Proteins. c. Fats. d. Minerals. e. Vitamins. f. Water.

34. c	39. d	44. c	49. d
35. c	40. a	45. d	50. d
36. c	41. c	46. d	51. a
37. b	42. c	47. a	52. c
38. c	43. a	48. c	53. d

Chapter 27   The Child Experiencing Surgery

1. a. Metabolic rate is much greater proportionately than that of adults; children need to be fed more frequently. b. Children lack physical reserves that are available to adults. their general condition can change very rapidly, almost without warning. Fluid intake and output must be calculated carefully. c. Body tissues of children heal quickly because of their rapid rate of metabolism and growth. d. Young children are more oriented to the present than to the future.

2. a. (1) Vocalization or cry. (2) Facial expression or grimace. (3) Body movement involving all four extremities. (4) Autonomic nervous system responses: increased pulse and BP, sweating, muscle tension, and gastrointestinal mobility. b. Any six of the following: (1) The development of trust. (2) Appropriate preparation for procedures. (3) Relaxation techniques. (4) Soothing presence and voice of parent or friend. (5) Guided imagery. (6) Hypnosis. (7) Distraction. (8) Play therapy. (9) TENS. (10) Repositioning. (11) Provision for rest. (12) Hot or cold applications. (13) Elevation of an injured part.

3. a. (1) Prevent nausea and vomiting. (2) Relieve postoperative abdominal distention and pressure or surgical repairs. b. To keep the tube patent; size of child, type of operation, and thickness of drainage. c. Low intermittent or gravity drainage.

4. a. Inject 1 to 5 cc of air while listening over the sternum for the characteristic sound. b. Withdraw the air and suction for stomach contents. c. Ask the patient to hum.

5. Any three of the following: a. Good hand washing. b. Not directly touching a soiled dressing. c. Touching inner dressings and wound areas with sterile gloves or forceps. d. Carefully disposing of old dressings. e. Changing dressings when they become damp.

6. b	10. b	14. d	18. a
7. c	11. a	15. b	
8. d	12. c	16. b	
9. b	13. a	17. c	

Chapter 28 Maintaining Oxygenation

1. a. Tongue. b. Trachea. c. Right bronchus. d. Diaphragm. e. Oral pharynx. f. Epiglottis. g. Larynx. h. Esophagus. i. Left bronchus. j. Bronchioles or secondary bronchi.

2. When ventilation of air into and out of the lungs is inhibited, the amount of oxygen available for cellular function is decreased.

3. An infant or child should be propped in a semi-Fowler's position or supported in an infant seat.

4. The child becomes cyanotic.

5. Any four of the following conditions: respiratory distress syndrome, aspiration, pneumonia, bronchiolitis, croup, asthma.

6. Any of the three following: headache, anxiety, agitation, confusion, weakness, double vision, and drowsiness.

7. Chemical analysis of oxygen and carbon dioxide levels in an arterial blood sample.

8. The Heimlich maneuver causes the diaphragm to suddenly force air out through the airway, which may dislodge the foreign body.

9. a. Catheter sizes vary with the size of the patient.
    b. Each patient has his own suction apparatus.
    c. Disposable drainage bottles.
    d. Catheters should be lubricated with saline or a water-soluble gel.
    e. Suction should be temporarily discontinued during insertion.
    f. Lowest amount of suction necessary should be intermittently applied and suction should not be prolonged.
    g. Catheter and connection tubing should be rinsed during and after use.
    h. Child may need to be restrained.
    i. Catheter should be discarded after use.
    j. Note should be taken of the type and amount of suctioned material obtained and the patient's tolerance of procedure.

10. A tracheostomy.

11. a. Explain use of signal cards or use of hand bells.
    b. Give the child a magic slate to write on.
    c. Give a pencil and paper to write on.
    d. Teach him to place his finger over the tracheostomy opening when he wants to talk or to use a tracheostomy plug.

12. To prevent infection.

13. In a well-ventilated room it is about 21%.

14. Blindness (retrolental fibroplasia).

15. Periodic blood gas determinations.

16. a. At least every 2 hours.
    b. No open flames should be allowed in the room and signs of "OXYGEN IN USE" should be clearly posted.
    c. Any electrical equipment used must be specially grounded to be safe.
    d. All enclosed oxygen units should be flushed with oxygen before patient is enclosed.
    e. To avoid carbon dioxide accumulation, all tents should provide some method of ventilation.

17. Incubators provide warmth, humidity, and easy observation of the infant.

18. If respiration has ceased and neck injury is not suspected, the child's head is tipped slightly more than in the "sniffing" or neutral position used with infants. The rescuer places his hand closest to the victim's head on the victim's forehead. The rescuer tilts the victim's head backward while using his other hand to raise the child's chin by placing his fingers against the bony jaw and lifting it upward. Two breaths 1 to 1.5 seconds are performed (mouth to mouth). Gentle breaths, just large enough to make the chest rise and fall. If a pulse is present, rescue breathing is continued at 15 ventilations/minute or every 4 seconds.

19. Resuscitation apparatus, suction setup, oxygen mask and cylinder, and emergency drug tray.

20. Use the typical head tilt and chin lift and/or oropharyngeal airway placement while also providing adequate support for the mask over the nose and mouth. The person providing ventilation may stand or sit behind the supine patient's head with the top of his head stabilized against her body. with one hand she holds the mask firmly against the patient's nose and mouth while maintaining his airway. With the other hand, she squeezes the air bag at a rate and depth compatible with the size and needs of the infant. The typical rate is the same as that used for mouth-to-mouth resuscitation—every 4 seconds.

21. It is less fatiguing for the operator and also helps to prevent possible disease transmission.

22. a. To treat hypoxemia and tissue hypoxia. b. To provide adequate ventilation for the child who cannot breathe on his own. c. To maintain positive pressure in the airways. d. To reduce the work of breathing.

23. a. Decrease or increase in normal resting respiratory rate. b. Noisy, labored breathing. c. Retractions. d. Flaring of nostrils. e. Pallor or cyanosis. f. Restlessness, apprehension, and disorientation. g. Thick respiratory tract secretions. h. Frequent coughing.

24. b 27. c 30. a 33. b
25. c 28. c 31. a
26. b 29. d 32. a

EXERCISE IX   CHILD HEALTH PROBLEMS

Chapter 29 Alterations in Body Temperature

1. Brings comfort; helps to avoid complications that occur in the presence of high fever or abnormal loss of body heat.

2. 97.6° F (36.4° C) to 99° F (37.8° C).

3. A balance between heat production and heat loss in the body.

4. Activity of all cells made possible by oxidation or burning of foodstuff within those cells.

5. By blood flowing through various parts of the body.

6. a. Involuntary constriction of blood vessels of the skin, thus forcing more blood into the warm interior of the body and cutting it off from cooler areas near the skin's surface. b. Automatic reduction of perspiration. c. Adding clothing to the body. d. Involuntary contraction of muscles—"shivering."

7. Hypothalamus.

8. The temperature regulation mechanism is immature or not perfected.

9. May help to fight infection and support the immune system, warns the individual of the presence of a possible disease process.

10. Convulsions.

11. a. Evaporation by failure to dry an infant during a bath or immediately following birth. b. Conduction by his contact with cold examining tables or scales. c. Convection by his exposure to drafts, cool oxygen flow (especially over his face). d. Radiation by his proximity to cold walls or other large objects.

12. To conserve calories, avoiding weight loss and acidosis.

13. For patients undergoing cardiac or thoracic surgery.

14. c	18. a	22. b	26. c
15. d	19. a	23. c	27. d
16. c	20. b	24. b	28. d
17. c	21. d	25. c	

Chapter 30 Skin Problems

1. Principally through capillary dilation and constriction and formation of cooling perspiration.

2. b, e, a, c, d.

3. a. Size. b. Elevation. c. Quality. d. Color. e. Distribution. f. Associated sensory disturbances. g. Type of exudate.

4. a. Poorly washed diapers. b. Infrequent diaper changes. c. Prolonged use of plastic diaper covers. d. Incomplete washing of the diaper area.

5. a. Use of antiseptic diaper rinse. b. Careful washing and drying of diaper area.

6. Considered to be the most frequent manifestation of allergy in infancy.

7. By ingestion, inhalation, or contactants.

8. There is often a family history of some type of allergy.

9. Identify the offending allergens.

10. Any eight of the following: a. Plants. b. Drapes. c. Rugs. d. Fuzzy toys. e. Feathers. f. Wool blankets. g. Pets such as a house dog or cat. h. Mattress. i. Clothes hanging in the closet.

11. An oatmeal preparation that helps remove the crusts present on her skin and reduce pruritus.

12. Too many washings can cause the baby's skin to become dry. Such dryness should be avoided. A soap substitute is regularly used, and before Amber leaves the hospital the doctor will explain what product is best for Amber.

13. To prevent Amber from scratching and possibly infecting her skin lesions, since infants are readily susceptible to infections.

14. Perhaps when she is sleeping.

15. Amber should be immunized so that she is protected against the common but serious childhood diseases. The immunizations include DTP and OPV, Hib and Hepititis B vaccines.

16. Any two of the following: a. Hot coffee. b. Hot water in bathtubs. c. Pulling down electric frying pans on themselves.

17. a. Playing with matches. b. Using kerosene.

18. a. First degree (partial thickness) involves only the epidermis. It is very superficial; a tender, slightly swollen redness results. An example is the typical summer sunburn.
    b. Second degree (superficial) involves the epidermis and dermis; it can be either superficial or deep. Deep burns may be converted from partial-thickness to full-thickness wounds by infection, trauma, or obliteration of the blood supply to the affected part. A second-degree burn is characterized by blister formation or a reddened, discolored region with a moist, weeping surface.
    c. Third degree (full thickness) involves the entire dermis and portions of the subcutaneous tissue. The region effectuate has a brown, leathery appearance with little surface moisture.

19. If water is readily available, it should be used; if not, handy blankets or throw rugs can be employed to smother the flames. If neither is available, the victim should be rolled on the ground or floor.

20. The burned area should be rinsed immediately with cold water if possible; quickly transport the child, wrapped in a clean sheet and blanket.

21. a. Maintain airway. b. Prevent shock.

22. Need for asepsis in caring for any burn patient. Everyone caring for individuals with serious burns must wear masks.

23. He is given nothing by mouth because he may go to surgery. A nasogastric tube may be inserted to prevent the onset of gastric dilation and paralytic ileus.

24. The amount and type of urine formation per hour.

25. Tetanus toxoid. b. Strict isolation. c. Penicillin.

26. Full-thickness burns usually leave no nerve endings intact.

27. In the operating room, with the patient under hypotensive anesthesia, which minimizes bleeding, devitalized burned tissue is cut away to the fascia, and skin grafts are immediately applied.

28. These biologic dressings are used to cover the wound and prevent infection in preparation for skin autografts.

29. b	35. c	41. c	47. c
30. d	36. a	42. b	48. a
31. c	37. b	43. b	49. c
32. b	38. a	44. a	50. c
33. d	39. c	45. b	
34. a	40. b	46. c	

Chapter 31   Infectious Disorders

1. h, f, c, e, d, g, b, a.

2. To provide for the safety of patients, visitors, students, and staff.

3. Knowledge of how a contagious disease is transmitted or the chain of infection.

4. a. Keeps records of rates of infection. b. Proposes investigations to determine reasons for difficulty in patient care practices associated with infection risk. c. Conducts examinations of appropriate interventions to reduce those risks. d. Helps interpret and prepare protocols for many hospital practices, including isolation precautions. e. Consultant and educational resource.

5. Epidemiology.

6. Second phase, called prodrome.

7. Reservoir of infectious agents.

8. The person who is in the second phase of the incubation period.

9. a. Free of communicable infections. b. Knowledgeable regarding possible special need to reevaluate assignment. c. Maintains good general health habits. d. Knowledgeable and dependable regarding infection precautions needed.

10. a. Proper nutrition. b. Adequate rest. c. Good personal hygiene. d. Use of stress reduction techniques.

11. Hand washing is a vigorous systematic rubbing together of all surfaces of lathered hands (usually lasting 10 seconds or more), followed by rinsing under a stream of water. Care should be taken not to recontaminate hands on faucets or other equipment.

12. a. A sink, running water, and a toilet. b. Box of gloves. c. Antimicrobial detergent. d. Paper towels. e. Laundry hamper. f. Plastic bags for trash. g. Gowns and masks if needed.

13. The type of isolation technique ordered and the visitor and patient being considered.

14. a. Direct, indirect, and droplet contact. b. Airborne. c. Common vehicle. d. Vector-borne.

15.

Disease	Infectious agent	Mode of transmission	Communicable period	Incubation period	Prevention
Bacillary dysentery	Shigella sonnei (most common), Shigella dysenteriae Shigella flexneri	Direct or indirect contact with feces of infected patients or carriers, contaminated water or food, flies	As long as patients or carriers harbor organisms (as determined by stool or rectal cultures)	1 to 7 days, usually 2 to 4	Attack may confer limited immunity; improve individual and community hygiene
Chickenpox (Varicella)	Varicella-zoster virus; primary response	Direct or indirect contact with respiratory secretions or moist skin lesions	1 to 2 days before rash until 6 days after its onset; dried crusts not contagious	10 to 21 days, usually 14	Immune after 1 attack. OKA vaccine for high-risk patients. VZIG can prevent or modify the course of disease when given shortly after exposure.
Rubella	Rubella virus	Direct contact with secretions from nose and mouth; may be acquired in utero	1 week before rash until 7 days after onset	14 to 21 days, usually 18	Rubella vaccine; immune after 1 attack
Measles	Measles virus	Direct or indirect contact with secretions from nose and throat, perhaps airborne; may be acquired in utero	From time of cold symptoms until 4 days after rash appears	8 to 12 days	Live measles vaccine; IG will prevent or modify disease if given within 6 days of exposure; immune after 1 attack

15. (continued)

Disease	Infectious agent	Mode of transmission	Communicable period	Incubation period	Prevention
Meningococcal meningitis	Neisseria meningitidis	Direct contact with patient or carrier by droplet spread	As long as organism is present in nose; usually not infectious after 24 hours of antibiotic therapy	1 to 10 days, usually 4 or less	Meningococcal polysaccharide vaccines for groups A and C; extent of immunity after attack unknown; rifampin used prophylactically for intimate contact
Infectious mononucleous	Epstein-Barr virus	Droplets from nose and throat, saliva	Unknown	Unknown	No immunization
Mumps	Mumps virus (Paramyxovirus)	Direct or indirect contact with patient by droplet spread	Several days before infection, up to 9 days after onset	14 to 21 days, usually 18	Mumps vaccine; immune after 1 attack
Hepatitis (HAV)	Hepatitis type A virus	Person to person; oral-fecal routes	2 weeks before jaundice (uncertain)	15 to 50 days, average 28	One attack confers immunity; IG protects if given within 72 hours after exposure.

16. b	20. d	24. a	28. c	32. b
17. b	21. b	25. b	29. c	33. c
18. d	22. c	26. d	30. c	34. d
19. c	23. b	27. b	31. b	35. a

Chapter 32 Neurosensory and Musculoskeletal Disorders

1. a, c, b, d.

2. Any two of the following: a. Phenytoin (Dilantin). b. Phenobarbital. c. Carbamazepine (Tegretol). d. Valproate (Depakene). e. Ethosuximide (Zarontin). f. Clonazepam (Clonopin). g. Primidone (Mysoline). h. Clorazepate (Tranxene).

3. Any five of the following: a. Pressure on brain. b. Cerebral anoxia. c. Direct injury. d. Embolus. e. Hemorrhage. f. Arrested hydrocephalus. g. Infection of brain. h. Toxicity of brain.

4. a. Kyphosis (humpback). b. Lordosis (exaggerated lumbar curvature). c. Scoliosis (S-shaped lateral curvature).

5. a. Poliomyelitis. b. Duchenne muscular dystrophy. c. Myelomeningocele. d. Other neuromuscular disorders.

6. a. Observation of voiding, stool, dressing. b. Respiratory symptoms. c. Neurologic symptoms.

7. a. Careful positioning, straight back, log rolling as ordered. b. Neurologic observations. c. Deep breathing, turning, range of motion, skin care. d. Fluids increased.

8. An internal metal rod attached to the vertebral column to obtain and maintain spinal correction.

9. The Milwaukee brace is used in the nonoperative treatment of mild spinal curvatures. Prevention of progression of the curve is likely when treatment is begun early.

10. 1 year.

11. Upper middle part of Fig. 32-1, p. 649.

12. Lower left-hand part of Fig. 32-1, p. 649.

13. a. The fracture needed reduction. More weight was probably necessary than was available through skin traction. An open reduction might be performed.
    b. She would be able to raise up with the use of an overhead bar and trapeze; could sit up in bed periodically; could turn slightly toward the broken leg while supine.
    c. Any six of the following: (1) Good position. (2) to breathe and cough deeply. (3) Skin care. (4) Infection, neurological, and circulation checks. (5) Observation of traction device. (6) Increased fluid intake. (7) Check of constipation. (8) Psychological stimulation.

14. Side rails; padded crib sides.

15. Turn her to her side. Keep her from injury, but do not restrain.

16. a. When the seizure began and what immediately preceded it. b. How the seizure progressed. c. Position of the eyes. d. How long the attach lasted. e. The need for suctioning or oxygen.

17. No; it is subjective.

18. Involuntary, uncoordinated, purposeless movements involving joint rather than single muscle action. The upper extremities are more often involved.

19. a. Pediatrician. b. Orthopedist. c. Physical therapist. d. Occupational therapist. e. Speech therapist. f. Psychologist. g. Medical-social worker. h. Public health worker. i. Nurse. j. School teacher.

20. 20.

21. Almost all the time except for brief periods devoted to hygienic care or special ordered exercise.

22. a	29. a	36. d	43. b	50. c
23. d	30. a	37. d	44. a	51. c
24. a	31. b	38. b	45. b	52. b
25. b	32. c	39. a	46. c	53. b
26. a	33. d	40. c	47. b	54. d
27. c	34. b	41. c	48. c	55. c
28. a	35. a	42. d	49. a	

Chapter 33   Orthopedic Technology

1. a. Reduce a fracture. b. Reduce a dislocated hip. c. Prevent and treat contracture deformities. d. Relieve muscle spasm and pain.

2. Skin traction helps position the bone indirectly by pulling on the skin and muscles. It is relatively simple to apply and involves no surgical operation.

3. a. Can be irritating to the skin. b. Supportive wrapping may cause allergic reactions or circulation or friction difficulties.

4. By inserting some mechanical device, such as wires, pins, or tongs, directly into or through bone and attaching prescribed weight.

5. a. Since bone is pierced, there is always danger of infection; a surgical procedure is involved in both insertion and removal. b. Area of insertion must be frequently inspected for signs of inflammation, infection, and drainage.

6. Pull in one direction must be balanced by pull in the opposite direction (counteraction) for traction to be effectively maintained.

7. a. Manual maintenance of body position. b. Elevation of the part of the bed next to the weights. c. Use of restraints. d. Application of a counterweight.

8. No traction or change in the angle of pull, which can distort the desired result.

9. Any five of the following: a. Keep bed linen smooth and tight. b. Eliminate any crumbs or other irritating small objects from the bed. c. Frequently inspect and cleanse susceptible body areas and use eggcrate mattress or sheepskin sheets. d. Use an overhead bar and trapeze to facilitate frequent attention to back care and skin care. e. Use lamb's wool under the patient. f. Apply tincture of Benzoin to bony prominences that are not red.

10. To promote continued traction as well as mobilization, a cast is placed over a skeletal traction pin.

11. Plaster of Paris<n>impregnated crinoline bandages that have been applied and molded while moist over some type of soft protective layer and allowed to dry to a hard resistant shell. Fiberglass and other plastic materials are now being used more frequently.

12. This depends on his rate of growth, condition of cast, and progress of desired correction.

13. Any six of the following: a. Puffiness. b. Pallor. c. Purple tint. d. Pressure response delay. e. Pulselessness. f. Paralysis. g. Paresthesia. h. Pain.

14. Pressure is made on nail beds to blanch area. When pressure is removed, normal nail color should return immediately.

15. Note time, and mark original size of stain with a pencil; check it often.

16. Every 2 to 3 hours.

17. Furnish support, maintain position, and provide strength to a body part.

18. In the supine position the patient extends and adducts his legs while wearing the shoes he will be using when walking. the nurse can measure from the patient's axilla to a point 4 to 8 inches out from his heel. If such positioning is difficult, the nurse can subtract 16 inches from the patient's height. Measurements must also consider the condition of the patient and the gait to be used.

19. Hands.

20. Any five of the following: a. Bed board to prevent mattress from sagging. b. Several firm plastic-covered pillows to support cast in position. c. Possibly an overhead bar and trapeze attached to the bed. d. Cast drier or well-ventilated room. e. A fracture pan. f. Cast board if available and appropriate plastic strips to protect perineal area. g. Urine-collecting bag to protect cast.

21. 24 hours.

22. When a chalky white finish and hard, nonmoist surface develops.

23. By petaling the edges of the cast.

24. Application of water-repellent adhesive strips cut to fit around perineal edge and other rough edges of the cast.

25. Cast can be cleaned with a damp, not wet, cloth and some type of white cleanser, such as Bon Ami, or fast-drying white shoe polish can be applied.

26. a	28. b	30. a	32. d
27. d	29. b	31. c	33. b

Chapter 34 Respiratory and Cardiovascular Disorders

1. b, d, e, a, f, g, c.

2. a. (1) Pneumococcal. (2) Staphylococcal. (3) Streptococcal. (4) *Haemophilus influenzae*.
   b. (1) viral. (2) *Mycoplasma*.

3. a. Fever. b. Anorexia. c. Listlessness. d. Cough.

4. Rapid and shallow, accompanied by flaring of nostrils, grunting, and retractions.

5. a. Cyanosis. b. A rapid, weak pulse.

6. a. WBC and differential blood count. b. Tracheal cultures. c. X-ray film.

7. Pneumococcal.

8. Pneumococcal.

9. a. Unable to take fluids, b. Need oxygen therapy. c. Surgical drainage indicated. d. Family not able to care for child.

10. a. Superior vena cava. b. Inferior vena cava. c. Right atrium. d. Tricupsid valve. e. Right ventricle. f. Pulmonary valve. g. Pulmonary artery. h. From lungs via pulmonary veins. i. Left atrium. j. Bicuspid or mitral valve. k. Left ventricle. l. Aortic valve. m. Aorta. n. Descending aorta. o. Myocardium.

11. a. Occurs when more blood than normal enters a ventricle. b. Results when outflow of blood is impeded or slowed. c. Low oxygen concentration of circulating arterial blood, which results from mixing of unoxygenated blood returning from the body with oxygenated blood returning from the lungs.

12. Acidosis and cyanosis.

13. a. Manifested by blueness of lips, nail beds, and mucosal surfaces. May be the result of shunting of unoxygenated blood into the left side of the heart or may be associated with pulmonary edema.
    b. A resting respiratory rate of about 50 per minute in the full-term infant or over 60 per minute in the premature. Symptoms are flaring of nostrils and rapid breathing.
    c. A heart rate greater than 180 beats per minute at rest.
    d. Chiefly manifested by feeding problems; infant becomes easily fatigued, stops nursing, and seldom finishes a bottle.
    e. Failure to gain weight.
    f. Murmurs or abnormal heart sounds that occur when the walls of vessels are uneven, valvular surfaces are irregular, or congenital defects are present.

14. Congestive heart failure.

15. d, b, e, c, a.

16. Pressure in various areas of the cardiocirculatory system and the percentage of oxygen in different chambers and great vessels.

17. Soon after birth, within a few weeks.

18. Oxygenated blood flows from the aorta back to the pulmonary artery for a return trip to the lung. This increases the workload on the left ventricle, can cause poor physical development, and decreases exercise tolerance and often life expectancy as a result of pulmonary vascular resistance.

19. a. Innominate. b. Left carotid. c. Left subclavian arteries.

20. Narrowing of aorta.

21. Pulses are weak or absent.

22. a. Headache. b. Leg cramps. c. Possible excessive fatigue. d. Frequent nosebleeds.

23. The narrowed portion of the aorta is cut out, and adjoining segments are sutured together. Occasionally repair involves insertion of a prosthesis.

24. Volume overload.

25. Left-to-right shunt is reversed, and a cyanotic condition results.

26. a. Decreased resistance to infections of the upper respiratory tract. b. Lowered exercise tolerance. c. Physical underdevelopment.

27. Yes, but if the opening is very large, incorporation of a plastic patch in the repair may be necessary.

28. Depends on the position and size of the defect and the presence of any abnormalities in the heart or great vessels.

29. Acyanotic.

30. Shunt is reversed, and the child becomes cyanotic.

31. Surgical repair by open heart surgery.

32. a. Interventricular septal defect. b. Pulmonary stenosis. c. Overriding aorta. d. Right ventricular hypertrophy.

33. The child typically has blue lips and nail beds and dusky-tinted skin, which becomes more cyanotic on exertion. He is likely to be small for his age.

34. The infant or child may have "hypoxemic spells" with respiratory distress, which cause deep cyanosis, loss of consciousness, and even convulsions.

35. This position improves oxygenation to the upper portion of his body by trapping some of the desaturated blood in the lower extremities.

36. Open heart surgery offers a chance for total correction.

37. Staphylococcal pneumonia often spreads to the lungs via the bloodstream from a staphylococcal infection elsewhere in the body.

38. His pneumonia is probably complicated by the formation of abscesses or pneumothorax.

39. Nafcillin sodium or oxacillin sodium.

40. A few weeks.

41. Because pneumococcal pneumonia is most common, therapy for all pneumonias is typically begun with penicillin, which is specific for this type; when culture results are obtained, specific therapy is initiated.

42.

Problems	Intervention
Fever 102° F	Rest, cool environment, fluids, and acetaminophen (Tylenol) as ordered
Viscid secretions	Humidification and increased fluids, deep breathing or laughing; chest physical therapy and suction.
Anorexia	Clear nasal passage before feeding; fluids should be encouraged.
Dyspnea and flaring nostrils	Infant seat; oxygen as ordered.

43. c	53. b	63. d	73. b	83. c
44. b	54. a	64. c	74. c	84. d
45. d	55. a	65. a	75. b	85. b
46. c	56. c	66. c	76. a	86. c
47. a	57. d	67. a	77. d	87. a
48. c	58. d	68. d	78. b	88. d
49. a	59. c	69. d	79. d	89. b
50. c	60. b	70. b	80. c	90. c
51. d	61. b	71. a	81. b	91. d
52. b	62. b	72. a	82. d	92. a

Chapter 35   Gastrointestinal and Metabolic Problems

1. Mechanical digestion takes place through the action of the teeth, tongue, cheeks, and muscular contractions called peristalsis. Chemical digestion takes place through the action of various enzymes, emulsifiers, acids, and bacteria that are normally active in different portions of the tract.

2. Any six of the following: a. Anorexia. b. Nausea. c. Vomiting. d. Constipation. e. Diarrhea. f. Weight loss. g. Abdominal distention.

3. Antibiotics destroy normal flora of the alimentary canal and allow the fungus to multiply without competition.

4. The exact etiology of diabetes mellitus is not known, but inheritance plays an important role.

5. a. Children are more likely to have a more abrupt onset of the disease than adults, who tend to develop diabetes gradually. b. As the condition progresses, the islets atrophy, finally becoming entirely incapable of insulin production. (Children are almost always insulin-dependent).

6. Detection of glycosuria together with the finding of an elevated blood glucose level (hyperglycemia) and ketonuria. No further tests are necessary.

7. e, g, c, d, b, a, f.

8. The nutritional intake should be comparable to that of a nondiabetic healthy child of the same age, sex, weight, and activity.

9. a. Growth b. Activity c. Appetite d. Culture e. Socioeconomic status f. Sensitivity to ethnicity.

10. a. Common foods should be used that can be modified to meet the tastes and economic needs of the child and family.
    b. On regularity of food intake and avoidance of simple sugars.

11.

◆◆◆ TYPES OF INSULIN

Type	Onset of action	Peak action (hours after injection)	Effective duration in hours
Regular	1/2 to 1 hr	2 to 4	6 to 8
Semilente	1/2 to 1 hr	2 to 4	8 to 10
Globin	1 to 2 hr	6 to 8	12 to 14
NPH	1 to 2 hr	6 to 8+	12 to 14
Lente	1 to 2 hr+	6 to 12+	14 to 16

12. The insulins should be drawn up in the same syringe and always in the same sequence; begin with short-acting, so that any residual insulin in the "dead space" remains constant.

13. When a child's condition is being regulated in the hospital, he is often placed on "regular insulin coverage," which means that the amount of insulin he receives depends on the amount of blood sugar and the presence or absence of urinary ketones.

14. General malaise; nausea, vomiting; abdominal pain; long, deep, labored respirations; "apple pie" breath, red lips; dehydration; low BPs; rapid, thready pulse; and irritability, drowsiness, coma, and death.

15. Fatigue, weakness, faintness, irritability, and personality changes; hunger; pale, clammy skin, diaphoresis; lethargy, and semiconscious state; and tumors, convulsions, and death.

16. A preparation available in a 1 mg vial for subcutaneous or intramuscular use. Glucagon activates liver enzymes and breaks down liver glycogen to produce glucose. It can be given when a child manifests signs of insulin reaction. It must be remembered, however, that it takes 10 to 20 minutes to work, and the child should be fed immediately.

17. a. You should first explain how to collect a blood specimen by using an automatic finger pricking device. If the Accu Chek IIm is used, the nurse should carefully read the directions with Cindy and be sure that she understands how to follow the directions. the manufacturer's directions must be followed, especially the "timing" during the procedure.
    b. Thirty minutes before breakfast and the morning insulin, and 30 minutes before dinner and the evening insulin.

18. Yes, most babies have a good appetite because the defect consists of a narrowing of the pyloric sphincter, which forms the exit of the stomach and therefore does not interfere with appetite.

19. Oscar has not gained any weight in 1 week's time. If the condition progresses, he will soon display a marked loss in weight.

20. During this operation the surgeon cuts down through the enlarged muscle of the pylorus to the mucous membrane. This relieves the constriction and is highly successful in relieving the cause of persistent vomiting.

21. If Oscar can keep down his feedings of glucose water after surgery, he will rapidly progress to half-strength formula and finally to his regular formula. If all goes well and Oscar retains his formula, he can be discharged as early as the same day following surgery.

22. A telescoping of the bowel that usually involves the ileocecal valve.

23. The pressure of the inflowing enema can reduce intussusception, but may have to be repeated more than once.

24. b	28. c	32. b	36. a
25. c	29. a	33. c	37. c
26. a	30. c	34. c	38. a
27. b	31. d	35. c	

Chapter 36   Genitourinary Problems

1. a. Kidney. b. Ureter. c. Bladder. d. Urethra. e. Ureter. f. Renal pelvis. g. Calyx. h. Cortex. i. Fibrous capsule. j. Medulla, k. Nephron. l. Artery. m. Glomerulus. n. Bowman's space. o. Proximal convoluted tubule. p. Loop of Henle. q. Distal convoluted tubule. r. Collecting duct. s. Secondary capillary network. t. Vein.

2. a. Filtration. b. Reabsorption. c. Secretion.

3. c, b, e, f, g, d, a.

4. a. Any three of the following: (1) Higher incidence of testicular malignancy. (2) Torsion. (3) Injury.
   b. (1) Injections of human chorionic gonadotropin. (2) Orchiopexy.

5. Hypospadias involves the termination of the urethra on the underside of the penis rather than at the normal site at its tip. The child avoids ridicule from his peers when surgical correction is done early.

6. a. Observation of the penile dressing for the amount and kind of drainage. b. Observation of the amount and type of urinary catheter drainage. c. Observation for any swelling.

7. The penis may show scars, but urinary and reproductive capacity is usually normal.

8. a. Evidence of reflux. b. Congenital structural defects that can impair urinary tract function.

9. The anatomic defect is repaired. The surgical procedure restores functional anatomy of the vesicoureteral junction, ideally by removing the cause of the infection and preventing serious renal impairment.

10. The suprapubic catheter helps drain the bladder; the ureteral catheters serve primarily as splints for the newly implanted ureters.

11. a. Ensure that drainage tubes remain patent, without tension, and well arranged for drainage. b. Measure output of each tube. c. Encourage fluid as allowed. d. Anticipate discomfort with appropriate measures and medications.

12. Excellent.

13. a. Albuminuria. b. Low serum albumin levels. c. High serum cholesterol levels.

14. Any six of the following: a. Weight. b. Abdominal girth measurement. c. Intake and output. d. Test of urine for albumin. e. Restriction of salty intake, promotion of nutrition. f. Protection from infection. g. Excellent skin care, positioning. h. Maintenance of morale.

15. Share the information that sometimes enuresis is caused by physical problems that can be treated. Recommend a visit to a urologist. Point out that Billy has been well motivated to stop but still is having problems. Mention that some medications can be helpful, as can supportive techniques such as decreasing evening fluids, waking to go to the bathroom, and less tension regarding the problem.

16. a	19. d	22. c	25. b	28. b
17. c	20. b	23. b	26. c	29. d
18. c	21. b	24. c	27. b	30. c

Chapter 37 Hematological Problems

1. Anemia

2. Hemoglobin

3. a. Dietary deficiency of iron. b. Acute or chronic blood loss. c. Impaired absorption of iron

4. a. Pallor of the mucous membrane. b. Irritability. c. Anorexia. d. Listlessness.

5. African-Americans.

6. Alteration in one amino acid on the hemoglobin chain.

7. Malaria.

8. Thalassemia.

9. The X chromosome.

10. Factor VIII.

11. A primary malignant disease of the bone marrow characterized by an abnormal increase of immature WBCs or undifferentiated blast cells.

12. The uncontrolled proliferation of leukemic cells prevents production and development of normal blood cells, which leads to infection, anemia, and bleeding.

13. Bone marrow aspiration analysis.

14. Nonwhite children.

15. a. Fever. b. Fatigue. c. Weight loss. d. Pallor. e. Bruises.

16. A complete remission.

17. a. Leukopenia. b. Thrombocytopenia. c. Anemia.

18. The length of the first remission. The longer the remission endures, the more optimistic the prognosis.

19. The duration of remissions has been increased by the addition of prophylactic therapy to the central nervous system. The use of radiation, intrathecal methotrexate, or both will enhance Debra's chance for a complete and long remission.

20. Suggest that she make an appointment to discuss information with Debra's physician, since every child responds individually. However, you could go on to say that a number of children have a long remission that lasts for years. Children in remission must have regular medical supervision which includes blood tests that reveal relapse or termination of remission.

21. c	24. b	27. d	30. b
22. d	25. c	28. c	31. d
23. a	26. b	29. d	32. a

EXERCISE X THE CHILD AND FAMILY WITH SPECIAL NEEDS

Chapter 38 Rehabilitation

1. The ability to perform those daily activities that are characteristic of the normal functions for one's age and culture.

2. To foster maximum growth, development, independence, and personal fulfillment within the limitations of the handicap.

3. a. Maintain a sense of trust. b. Protect from fear, frustration, and pain. c. Facilitate social interactions and contact with community.

4. a. An inpatient unit. b. An outpatient clinic. c. Community agencies.

5. Any six of the following: a. Skin problems—frequent inspection, turning, good positioning, massage, cocoa butter to bony prominences, special foam rubber or "egg carton" mattress, good dietary intake. b. Muscle wasting, contractures, ankylosis—range of motion, frequent turning, good positioning, c. Venous flow problems, thrombosis—frequent turning, good positioning, elastic stockings or Ace wraps to legs. d. Urinary problems—high fluid intake, clean intermittent catheterization q. 4 hours. e. Bowel problems—high fluid intake, dietary roughage(?), stool softeners, possible suppository regimen. f. Respiratory stasis—stimulate cough, deep breathing by suctioning, frequent turning and change in position, intermittent positive-pressure breathing, later possible spirometer regimen. g. Depression, disorientation—regular supportive routine, presence of calendar and clocks, verbal and tactile stimulation, contact with family and friends. h. Social and developmental delay—as recovery permits increased on-unit socialization, community and home passes, close communication and cooperation with family.

6. Keep patient totally non-weight-bearing (free of pressure) until redness disappears.

7. Thirty seconds every 20 to 30 minutes.

8. Check her bladder for distention (her head is already elevated). Autonomic dysreflexia.

9. Any two of the following: a. Entrance—steps. b. Bathroom—space to maneuver, is door wide enough? c. Bedroom—space to maneuver, is clothing within reach? d. Hallways—are they wide enough? e. Floor plan—stairways? one or two floors? f. Kitchen—height and location of cupboards and appliances.

10. Denial (shock and disbelief). You reply might be: "I know you would like her to—we all would—but she really cannot move her legs." (Answer should recognize his feelings, reinforce reality, but not confront.)

11. b, b, a, a, b, a, c, c, a.

12. c	16. c	20. a	24. b
13. c	17. a	21. c	25. a
14. b	18. b	22. c	26. b
15. c	19. c	23. d	27. a

Chapter 39   Grief and Loss

1. a. Numbness. b. Yearning and searching. c. Despair and disorganization. d. Hope and rebuilding.

2. Any two of the following: a. Psychosocial development. b. Cognitive development. c. Past experience d. Cultural background.

3. 9 years or older.

4. Children this age are bothered by the disease process and its treatment. Shortly before treatment tell him what to expect. Encourage Mark by telling him that you will stay with him during treatment. Encourage his parents to be there when Mark's bone marrow aspiration is finished.

5. Involvement of parents in the physical care of their child is extremely important in facilitating parental adaptation of the diagnosis and the situation in general. Parents usually want to be with their sick child and need to feel that they personally have done everything possible for him. Mark's parents should be encouraged to participate in his care whenever possible. They should not be asked to leave.

6. Guilt feelings about the child's condition are often manifested by "If only I had done this or that; if only I had notified the physician sooner." It is natural to express these feelings; they are usually a sign of normal grief. It is a stage in the gradual process of accepting a great loss.

7. You should know and understand the mourning process that all parents go through. The process of resigning themselves to an inevitable outcome usually begins before the child dies, and you must allow parents this period of mourning, which involves a concentration of interest and energies, self-examination, self-condemnation, and guilt. You should allow parents to voice their guilt, and reassure them by the gentle and understanding way you answer their questions.

8. Tell Mr. and Mrs. Grey that you will be close by and will watch over Mark while they are gone.

9. Tell the staff that Mr. and Mrs. Grey are in conference with Mark's physician and that you told them you would especially watch Mark. Ask a staff member to take on the assignment until you get back.

10. Ask one of them to step out of the room with you to see about Mark's food tray. Outside the room tell the parent that you have put Mark's tray aside until after his bone marrow procedure, which the doctor discussed in conference. Tell them that it is best to inform Mark just before the procedure what is to be done so he will not worry too much.

11. c	13. b	15. a	17. b	19. b
12. b	14. d	16. b	18. b	20. b

Appendix

Words often misspelled in charting

abdomen	equal	perineum
abdominal	excoriated	pHisoHex
abscess	extremity	popsicle
ache	gurney	purulent
appetite	hygiene	reddened
bruise	inflamed	regurgitated
catheterization	inflammation	respiration
cereal	intact	respiratory
circulation	irritable	rough
congested	itch	scrape
cries	lesion	site (place)
cry	lochia	stomach
dilated	massage	stretcher
dining room	mucous (adjective)	suction
douche	mucus (noun)	syringe
dyspnea	nausea	tincture
dyspneic	noisy	urine
edema	occasional	vagina
edematous	paroxysmal	vinegar
emesis	perineal	